✦SUPERFOOD✦
JUICES & SMOOTHIES

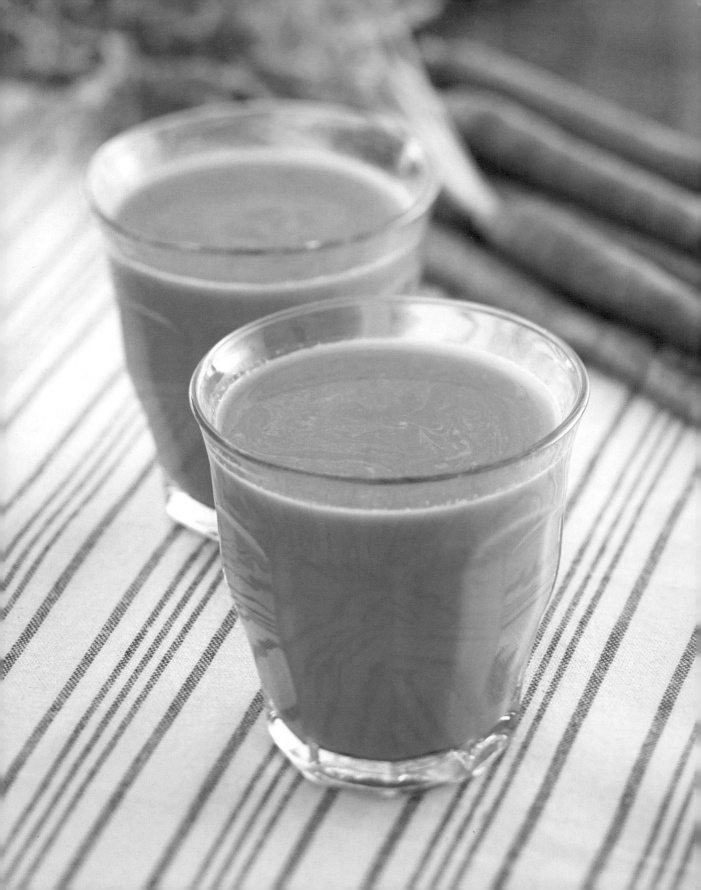

✦SUPERFOOD✦
JUICES & SMOOTHIES

100 Delicious and Mega-Nutritious Recipes from the World's Most Powerful Superfoods

By Tina Leigh, C.H.H.C.

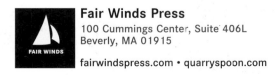

Fair Winds Press
100 Cummings Center, Suite 406L
Beverly, MA 01915

fairwindspress.com • quarryspoon.com

First published in the USA in 2014 by
Fair Winds Press, a member of
Quayside Publishing Group
100 Cummings Center
Suite 406-L
Beverly, MA 01915-6101
www.fairwindspress.com
Visit www.QuarrySPOON.com and help us celebrate food and culture one spoonful
at a time!

17 16 15 14 13   1 2 3 4 5

ISBN: 978-1-59233-604-3

Digital edition published in 2014
eISBN: 978-1-62788-019-0

Library of Congress Cataloging-in-Publication Data available

Cover and book design by Michelle Thompson/Fold & Gather Design
Interior layout by *tabula rasa* graphic design
Photography by Glenn Scott
Food styling by Jessica Weatherhead and Jennifer Beauchesne

Printed and bound in China

The information in this book is for educational purposes only. It is not intended to
replace the advice of a physician or medical practitioner. Please see your health care
provider before beginning any new health program.

CONTENTS

WHAT MAKES SUPERFOODS SUPER?

Goji, hemp, chia, flax, maca, cacao, wheatgrass! Ever wonder how or why these foods and others have received the esteemed "super" status when foods you would think are outrageously healthy don't receive such recognition? You're not alone. Many of those interested in superfoods are scratching their heads despite having heard common explanations such as these superfoods are nutrient-rich and considered to be especially beneficial for health and well-being. Many people still don't understand what it takes for these particular foods to receive such credit. I promise you, it's not because of an A-list celebrity fan base or that these foods are considered fashionable at the moment. There are legitimate reasons for them being labeled superfoods.

SUPERFOOD STARDOM GAINED FROM NUTRIENT DENSITY

The foremost reason a food is considered a superfood is because of nutrient density, which is the percentage of nutrients in a food compared to the number of calories. In the case of superfoods, the nutrient-to-calorie ratio falls disproportionately in favor of the nutrients, especially when compared to other healthy foods.

One system of measurement used to determine nutrient density is the Aggregate Nutrient Density Index, or ANDI. Joel Fuhrman, MD, author of *Eat for Health,* developed the ANDI in the late 1990s and later revised it in 2012. The ANDI evaluates twenty-three different nutrients within a single food, including antioxidants, minerals, vitamins, amino acids, and essential fatty acids. It then rates the food on a numbered scale from least (ANDI 0) to most (ANDI 1,000) nutritious. To demonstrate the density of a superfood compared to a non-super yet still healthy food, kale has an ANDI rating of 1,000 whereas a carrot has a rating of 336. Foods lacking in nutrition, such as graham crackers and soda, only score in the single digits.

Another system of measurement used by nutrition experts to classify foods is the Oxygen Radical Absorbance Capacity system, or ORAC. ORAC measures a food's ability to repel free radicals, a result of antioxidant activity. The higher the ORAC value, the greater the activity. To give you an idea of the kind of antioxidant power a superfood must demonstrate for it to be identified as such, an orange has an ORAC value of 3,000. Cherries weigh in at 3,700, blueberries at 6,500, but the goji berry, a well-known superfood, tops the charts at an ORAC value of 25,000! Staggering, don't you think?

SUPERFOODS AND PH BALANCE

In addition to their nutrient density, superfoods promote pH balance in the body. The term "pH," which stands for "potential of hydrogen," is a measurement of relative acidity and alkalinity; the body needs a balance of both for optimal health. The pH scale ranges from 0 to 14, with the acidic range being 0 to 6.9 and 7.1 to 14 considered alkaline. A measurement of 7 is considered neutral.

If our pH deviates too much from the ideal range of 7.35 to 7.45, our bodily systems begin to break down and we may begin to experience symptoms of inflammatory disease. In addition, as you will learn in the chapters that follow, diseased cells of any kind cannot thrive in an alkaline environment, and nearly all degenerative illnesses such as cancer, heart disease, and arthritis are associated with elevated acid levels in the body.

The foods we eat greatly influence changes in our pH levels. This is why it is essential we eat the most nutrient-dense foods possible, with a greater percentage of those being alkalinizing. The Western diet, for example, is considered highly acidic. But not all foods that seem acidic are, and you don't want to avoid them. Lemons are a great example of this. They taste acidic; however, when they meet enzymes in our body, they produce an alkalinizing effect on our pH levels. There are many resources online, one of which I have shared on page 197, which chart the acidity and alkalinity of different foods.

FOODS OF OUR ANCIENT ANCESTORS—SUPERFOODS OF TODAY

Nearly all superfoods that seem to have been recently discovered actually date back thousands of years. Goji berries, for example, have been cultivated and revered as promoting longevity among Asian cultures for more than three thousand years. South Americans have used chia and maca to stimulate energy levels, boost endurance, and promote a healthy sex drive since the days of the Incan and Aztec warriors.

Ancient inhabitants around the globe did not have the luxury of growing any food they wanted. Food was scarce, and people had to make do with their limited selection. That meant the few foods they could grow and consume had to contain the highest nutritive value possible. They needed their limited food supply to deliver all essential nutrients that support optimum health, strength, endurance, and vitality.

In addition, the food they cultivated needed to withstand the harshest of conditions, be it icy winter storms or extremely high elevations, such as in the Himalayas or the Andes. Many of the foods they grew were hearty, resilient, deeply nourishing, and have been on our planet for thousands of years. The staple foods of our ancient ancestors are the superfoods of our modern day, and how lucky we are to have such convenient access to them. Feel inspired to incorporate them into your diet? Good! It's time to try out twenty of my all-time favorites!

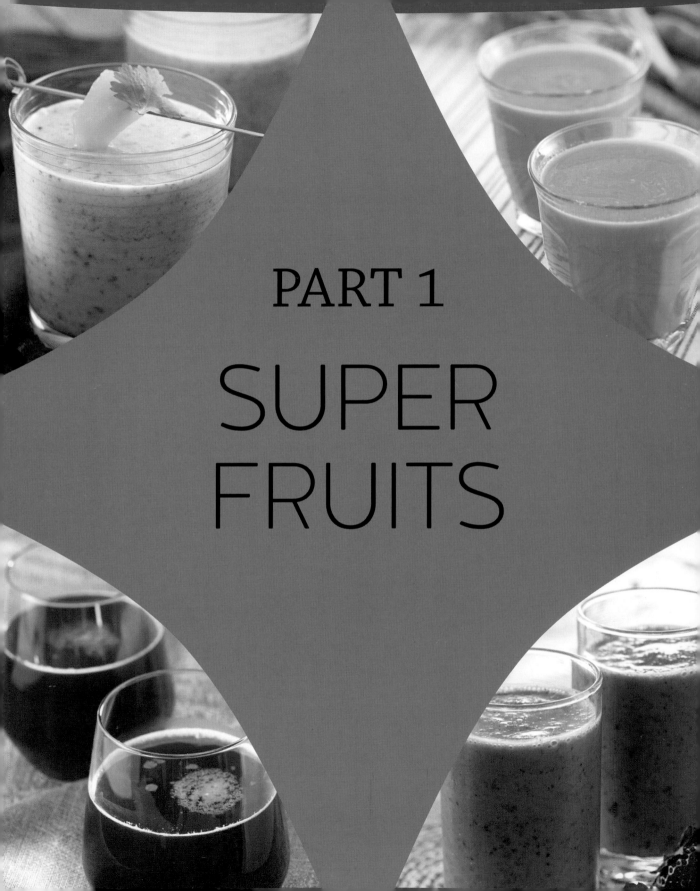

PART 1

SUPER FRUITS

CHAPTER 1

GOJI

THE "RED DIAMOND" OF NUTRITION

FEATURED RECIPES

Pure Goji Juice

Rosy Gems Juice

Liquid Sunshine Juice

Blush Smoothie

Chocolate Drop Smoothie

If it hasn't already, this delicate and nutritious berry will seduce you. Throughout Asia, goji berries (*Lycium barbarum*) are referred to as red diamonds not only for their beauty, but also their incredible nutritive properties.

These orangey-red berries have been enticing health-conscious eaters for years. You have likely seen them mixed into granola bars, smoothies, teas, trail mixes, cereals, salads, desserts, and chocolates. Their presence boosts the nutrient density of any food or beverage. They have also been popular in culinary circles for their distinct taste, one that produces a ravishing flavor fusion of smoke, salt, and tang. Goji's taste seamlessly complements bold flavors such as cacao, citrus, and vanilla.

ANTIOXIDANT WUNDERKIND

Goji berries have been around for thousands of years. The Tibetan and Chinese peoples were the initial cultivators of these wonder berries and revered goji as a life force food, believing it held the key to longevity. A double-blind placebo-controlled study published in 2008 in *The Journal of Alternative and Complementary Medicine* supports its purported health-giving properties, showing that a unique group of chemical compounds called *polysaccharides* contributed to the participants' increase in athletic and sexual performance, deeper sleep, and healthier gut function. A 2011 study by the same researchers published in *The Journal of the American College of Nutrition* showed that consumption of goji berries increased the metabolic rate and reduced the weight of test group subjects. Participants also reported enhanced feelings of well-being and an increase in energy.

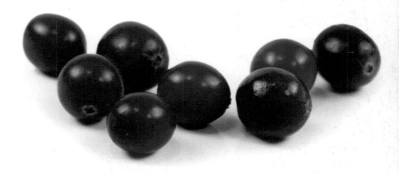

Diamonds Aren't Inexpensive

The most common form in which goji berries are enjoyed is dried. As mentioned before, they are sometimes referred to in commercial export as red diamonds, and they come with a proportionate price tag. Fortunately, they weigh very little, so if you can buy them in bulk, you'll save money. On average in America, ⅓ pound (150 g) costs $5.50 and equates to about 1¼ cups (135 g). That is actually a lot of goji as a suggested serving is 1 tablespoon (6 g). Also, 1¼ cups (135 g) dried berries makes about 80 ounces (2 L) of juice! So even though at first you may get sticker shock, it's not too bad when you consider the cost of each serving. And with its nutritional bang for the buck and culinary advantages, the cost is a bit more justifiable.

Goji berries also contain an astonishing level of antioxidants, which help fight damage caused by free radicals, atoms that contain an odd number of electrons. Why is this important? Atoms like to attach to bound pairs of electrons. Sometimes one electron breaks free, turning the formerly happy atom into an unstable free radical. Free radicals go wild, looking to steal an electron from a stable atom and turn them into free radicals, beginning the whole process over again.

Free radicals can attack cells and damage DNA, causing disease and oxidative stress, a sort of rusting from within that is similar to what happens when apple slices turn brown. Pollution, tobacco smoke, and an unhealthy diet all promote free radicals. The fight for healthy atom structure occurs all the time in the body, and when more energy is being spent on balancing the scales, less energy remains for healthy organ function.

Antioxidants are plant compounds that have the ability to slow oxidative stress, and goji berries are an antioxidant powerhouse. As stated in the introduction, they top the charts with an ORAC score of 25,000!

Goji berries also contain a high concentration of vitamin A and more vitamin C by weight than any other food on the planet except for camu camu berries, which are showcased in the next chapter. Also, noshing on 2 tablespoons (12 g) of dried goji berries delivers 20 percent of the recommended daily intake of iron. Iron is a vital nutrient that carries oxygen to your body's tissues, organs, and blood. You can become anemic when you have low iron levels. Symptoms of anemia include fatigue and muscle cramping. If you suspect or know you suffer from this condition, be sure to buddy up with the rosy goji to boost your intake of this essential mineral.

Even Good Things Have Side Effects

Goji is a member of the Solanaceae family, more commonly known as nightshade. If you have a known sensitivity to foods in this group, such as tomatoes, eggplant, peppers, and tomatillos, you may want to steer clear of them. The most notable symptoms of a nightshade sensitivity are abdominal cramps, diarrhea, achy joints, and headaches. In addition, those with pollen allergies may also experience adverse reactions when eating goji because of cross-contamination, so be sure you and pollen get along before adding goji berries to your diet.

Goji is also full of potassium, which is useful in a number of bodily functions. A 1-ounce (28 g) serving of the dried berries delivers 500 mg of potassium, roughly 25 percent of the suggested adult daily minimum. Potassium is best known for its promotion of balanced hydration in the body as well as healthy pituitary gland function. The pituitary gland produces human growth hormone (HGH), which naturally declines with age. Stimulating its production aids in reversing deterioration of our muscles and assists in fat burning and the tightening and toning of our skin.

And last, goji berries contain nearly 16 percent protein by dry weight! Impressive, don't you think?

IMMUNE-BOOSTING AND ANTI-INFLAMMATORY ACTION

Goji berries' polysaccharides are powerful immune boosters that promote the growth of healthy gut bacteria. Because most of our immune system resides in our gut, the more healthy gut flora we have, the more our immune system is being supported. A healthy immune system helps fight disease and viruses. This is why goji has developed a reputation for being a disease destroyer. Also, for thousands of years, inhabitants of Northern China have used goji medicinally to reduce inflammatory disease. They attribute a reduction in chronic pain, arthritis, asthma, and allergies to drinking goji tea. The Ningxia Hui region is where the majority of goji is grown and home to more centurions than the rest of the country. Goji is so revered by the people of this region that they hold a two-week festival every year in honor of its health benefits. The berry must be doing something right to earn that kind of recognition!

Sourcing and Care of Goji Berries

Goji powder is all the rage right now. This highly concentrated powder provides a convenient way to obtain the flavor and health benefits of goji berries in creamy desserts, juices, and smoothies. I like to use the vibrant reddish-orange powder for garnish by dusting a little on my smoothies. You can find the super powder in packages at your health food store.

When you buy goji berries, look for organic Tibetan varieties rather than Chinese wolfberries (their other name). The use of pesticides is common in Chinese production, and you don't want to negate all of the berries' healthful properties by eating those that have been grown conventionally.

Store your goji berries in an airtight glass container in a cool and dry environment such as your pantry. If you live in a humid climate, store in the refrigerator. In either case, dried goji berries will maintain strength in flavor and nutritive value for up to six months.

✦PURE GOJI JUICE✦

Making your own goji juice will save you money and result in pure, fresh, liquid gold rich with immune-boosting vitamin C and disease-fighting antioxidants. You also benefit from producing a tasty juice that doesn't have added sugar, an unnecessary additive often present in bottled varieties. The taste of this nutrient-rich juice is tangy and sweet and can be enjoyed alone or mixed into smoothies and juices.

Time: 8 to 12 hours (includes brewing time)

Equipment: 32-ounce (1 L) glass jar with a tight-fitting lid, blender, and fine-mesh strainer

Yield: Approximately 32 ounces (1 L)

Ingredients:
½ cup (45 g) goji berries
32 ounces (1 L) filtered water

Preparation:
Combine the goji berries and water in the glass jar. Apply the lid and let rest at room temperature for at least eight hours and ideally up to twelve.

Transfer the soaked berries and their liquid to a blender and purée on high for 1 minute.

Pour the juice back into the glass jar through a fine-mesh strainer. Store the juice in the refrigerator until ready to use. The juice will remain fresh for up to seven days.

✦ROSY GEMS JUICE✦

This fresh juice is especially healthful because of the addition of ginger. The root's phyto-compounds, *gingerols*, reduce inflammation in the body and support a reduction in joint and muscle aches. Lemon has a detoxifying effect by increasing liver function, and pectin from the apples supports healthy bowel function. The tartness of the apple enhances the smokey flavor of the goji juice. Fresh lemon adds vibrancy and makes it a refreshing beverage any time of day.

Time: 5 minutes

Equipment: Juicer

Yield: Approximately one 16-ounce (475 ml) juice

Ingredients:
1 handful fresh parsley

1 piece (½ inch, or 1 cm) fresh ginger

1 lemon, peeled with pith intact

1½ large tart apples (such as Fuji), halved

6 ounces (175 ml) Pure Goji Juice (see page 12)

Preparation:
Pass the parsley, ginger, lemon, and apples through a juicer. Transfer to a pint (475 ml) glass or jar and stir in the goji juice. Enjoy immediately and sip slowly.

✦LIQUID SUNSHINE JUICE✦

Think carrot juice on steroids! Carotenoids responsible for aiding in the prevention of cardiovascular disease and cancer are at an all-time high in this vibrant juice. Both carrots and goji berries are loaded with these powerful antioxidants. The combination of fresh orange and pure goji juices as well as sweet pressed carrot juice results in a delightfully creamy and nourishing tonic.

Time: 5 minutes

Equipment: Juicer

Yield: Approximately one 16-ounce (475 ml) juice

Ingredients:

½ lemon, peeled with pith intact

1 medium orange, peeled with pith intact

3 medium carrots, ends trimmed

6 ounces (175 ml) Pure Goji Juice (see page 12)

Preparation:

Pass the lemon, orange, and carrots through the juicer. Transfer to a pint (475 ml) glass or jar and stir in the goji juice. Enjoy immediately and sip slowly.

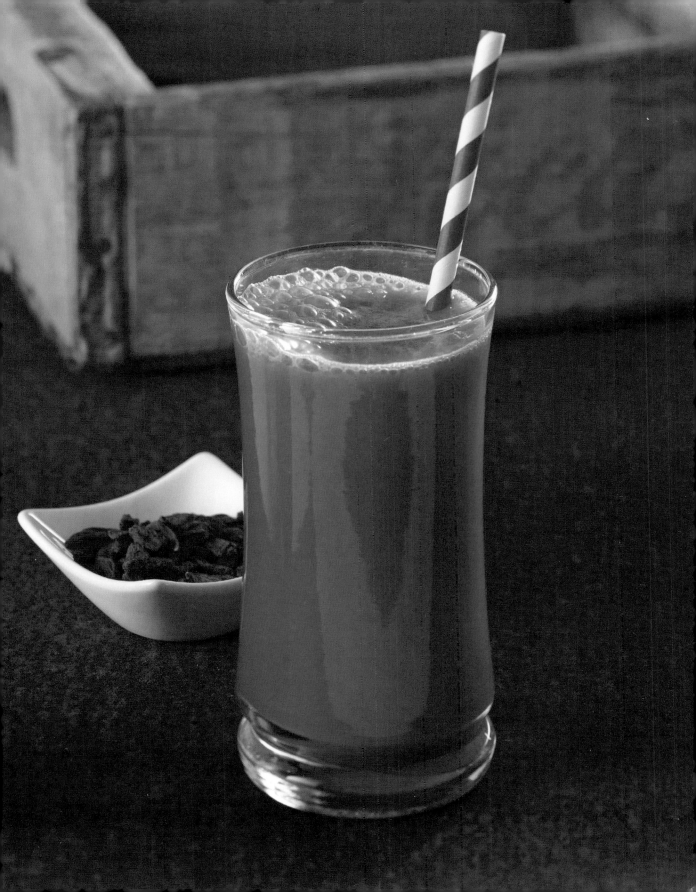

✦BLUSH SMOOTHIE✦

Enjoy this sweet and tangy anytime smoothie and reap the benefits of its nourishing ingredients. The dates, strawberries, and goji provide one-third of your recommended daily intake of fiber, and mint acts as a healthy digestive. The unusual combination of mint, orange, and goji imparts a refreshing flavor profile when blended with fresh or frozen strawberries. The balance of delicate flavors is so divine that even the strawberries blush.

Time: 5 minutes

Equipment: Blender

Yield: Approximately one 24-ounce (700 ml) smoothie

Ingredients:
1 cup (145 g) fresh or frozen strawberries

1 tablespoon (9 g) goji powder

1 heaping teaspoon orange zest

6 to 10 fresh mint leaves (to taste)

3 pitted medjool dates

1½ cups (355 ml) coconut or unsweetened almond milk

4 to 6 ice cubes (if using fresh strawberries)

Preparation:
In a blender, combine the strawberries, goji powder, orange zest, mint, dates, coconut or almond milk, and ice (if using fresh strawberries).

Blend on high for 20 seconds or until smooth.

Transfer to a large glass. Enjoy immediately and sip slowly.

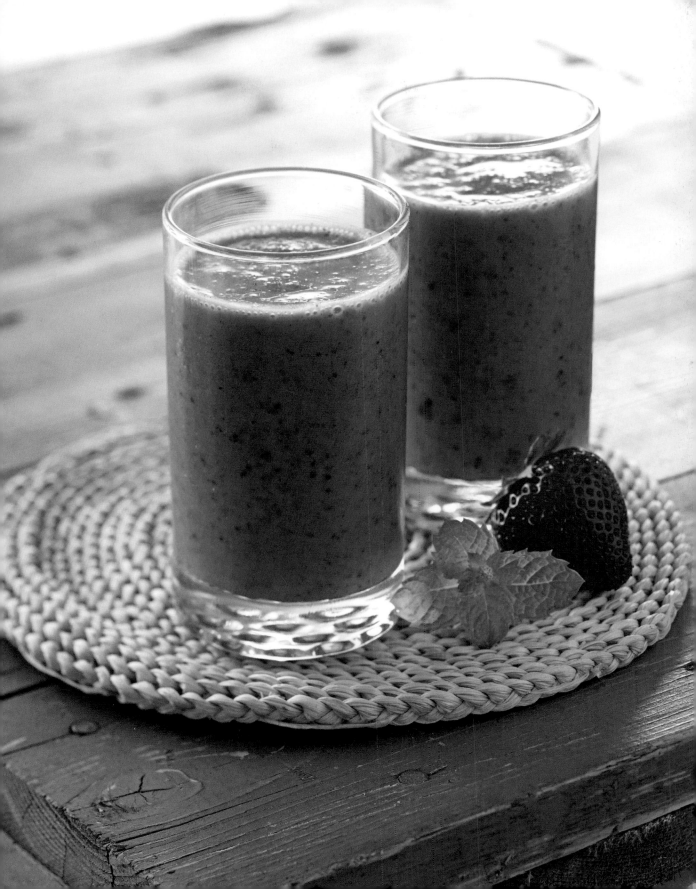

✦CHOCOLATE DROP✦ SMOOTHIE

Not only does this creamy smoothie taste like dessert, you get a mega-dose of disease-fighting compounds. The addition of raw cacao delivers an additional sixty-one antioxidants to the already abundant amount present in goji. You will also feel sated for hours from the inclusion of plant-based protein and fiber-rich avocado. The flavors of dark chocolate and goji are a match made in heaven. The smokiness and tang of the berries balance nicely with the bittersweet flavor of raw cacao. We are seeing this combination more and more in artisan chocolates and desserts. Whip up a little bit of decadence in a flash and indulge without guilt.

Time: 5 minutes

Equipment: Blender

Yield: Approximately one 24-ounce (700 ml) smoothie

Ingredients:

2 tablespoons (15 g) chocolate plant protein powder (such as pea or hemp)

¼ medium avocado, peeled and pitted

2 pitted medjool dates

1 tablespoon (9 g) goji powder

1½ cups (355 ml) coconut water

1 cup (235 ml) unsweetened almond milk

2 teaspoons (4 g) dried goji berries

Preparation:

In a blender, combine the protein powder, avocado, dates, goji powder, coconut water, and almond milk.

Blend on high for 20 seconds or until smooth.

Transfer to a large glass and garnish with dried goji berries. Enjoy immediately and sip slowly.

CHAPTER 2

CAMU CAMU

VITAMIN C SUPERSTAR

FEATURED RECIPES

Chocolate-Dipped Berry Smoothie
Sweetheart Juice
Glow Smoothie
Lemon Twist Smoothie
Pink Lemonade

You are sure to pucker up when this sour berry hits your pout. Like many of the super fruits that bless our food supply, the exotic camu camu is grown in the nutrient-rich rain forest soil of Peru and other hot and damp tropical climates. The plant bears cherry-sized berries that are highly acidic, very tart, and are often sweetened to please your palette. The camu camu berry contains one of the highest concentrations of vitamin C, a nutrient our body does not manufacture, but one that is essential for nearly three hundred functions.

THE POWER OF VITAMIN C IN PERSPECTIVE

The good ole' orange that has served as a common source of vitamin C for as long as we can remember contains, on average, 2,500 parts per million (ppm) of vitamin C. The camu camu berry's level of C towers over the orange at 50,000 ppm, or about 2 grams of the vitamin per 100 grams of fruit. Just 1 teaspoon of camu camu powder, the most common way to consume it, contains 1,180 percent of your recommended daily allowance (RDA), or 30 to 60 times more vitamin C than an orange. That's a lot of vitamin C!

Vitamin C, however, is not capable of supporting your well-being all on its own. You cannot take a vitamin C tablet and have it function as it does when ingested through whole foods. Why not? Because, to do its work efficiently, vitamin C must be delivered to our blood and cells in the company of other phytochemicals that are only present in plant foods such as fruits and vegetables.

CALM YOUR NERVES WITH VITAMIN C

The health of your brain and the intricate web of nerves in your body heavily rely on vitamin C for support. The way in which this antioxidant offers

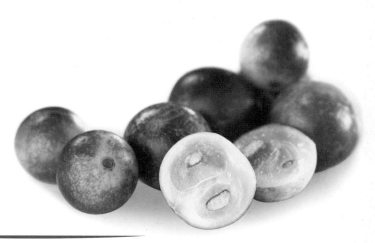

REDUCE INFLAMMATION WITH VITAMIN C-RICH FOODS

In 2008, four researchers from the Department of Cardiovascular and Renal Medicine at Saga University Faculty of Medicine in Japan set out to assess the anti-inflammatory properties of the camu camu berry. They engaged twenty male smokers with elevated oxidative stress. The smokers were each asked either to drink 70 ml (2 ½ ounces) of pure camu camu juice, which has a vitamin C concentration of 1,050 mg, or take the equivalent vitamin content in tablet form. The participants were studied for seven days. The results indicated that at the end of the week, oxidative stress markers such as C reactive protein, an indicator of cancer risk, had significantly declined in the group drinking camu camu juice, whereas there was no change in oxidative stress markers in those who took the tablets. This study affirms how essential it is not only to get ample vitamin C, but to do so by eating whole foods that contain vitamin C–supporting antioxidants and phytochemicals.

a helpful hand is by converting amino acids such as tryptophan and tyrosine to neurotransmitters like serotonin and dopamine. These mood-enhancing hormones help with focus, regulate learning, support restful sleep, and reduce anxiety and depression. When deficient in vitamin C, according to Victoria J. Drake, PhD, at Oregon State University, you may experience nerve-related disorders such as depression or even scurvy if left untreated.

In the medical journal *Sub-cellular Biochemistry*, published by the National Library of Medicine in 2012, a researcher at Vanderbilt University in Nashville stated that vitamin C protects neurons from oxidative damage, which is cellular stress that contributes to neurodegenerative disease such as Alzheimer's and Parkinson's.

So next time you are feeling like your head is in the clouds or if fog is hovering over you, instead of reaching for a stimulant such as caffeine or sugar, blend up a smoothie made with camu camu berries and enjoy a natural and antioxidant-rich high.

✦CHOCOLATE-DIPPED✦ BERRY SMOOTHIE

You will feel as though you've died and gone to heaven when the taste of this seductively sweet, tart, and chocolaty treat graces your lips. What's even more fantastic is you can enjoy this level of decadence without the guilt. The vitamin C in strawberries promotes elasticity of your skin and boosts collagen production. Can you say "natural wrinkle eraser?" Spinach and kale deliver calcium, magnesium, and vitamin K, all of which support the growth and strength of your bones. The combination of these body-beautifying and nurturing foods deliver a flavor that is simply intoxicating.

Time: 5 minutes

Equipment: Blender

Yield: Approximately one 20-ounce (570 ml) smoothie

Ingredients:

8 fresh or frozen strawberries

2 large kale leaves, de-ribbed and chopped

1 small handful spinach

3 tablespoons (23 g) chocolate plant protein powder (such as pea or hemp)

½ teaspoon camu camu powder

1½ cups (355 ml) unsweet- ened almond milk

8 ice cubes

Preparation:

In a blender, combine all the ingredients.

Blend on high for 20 seconds. Enjoy immediately and sip slowly.

✦SWEETHEART JUICE✦

Tangy, succulent, and full of nutrients, this juice will leave you puckering in delight. Red beet oxygenates and purifies your blood, while grapefruit and camu camu powder deliver immune-boosting and mood-enhancing vitamin C. Ginger reduces inflammation in the body and aids in digestion. The apple provides a sweet balance to the juice and delivers nutrients that nourish the gut and support healthy elimination.

Time: 10 minutes

Equipment: Juicer

Yield: Approximately one 16-ounce (475 ml) juice

Ingredients:
1 piece (½ inch, or 1 cm) fresh ginger

1 medium Ruby Red grape-
    fruit, peeled, with pith
    intact, quartered

1 medium red beet, trimmed
    and halved

2 medium sweet apples (such
    as Red Delicious), halved

½ teaspoon camu camu powder

Preparation:
Pass the ginger, grapefruit, beet, and apples through a juicer in the order specified.

Transfer to a serving glass and garnish with camu camu powder. Enjoy immediately and sip slowly.

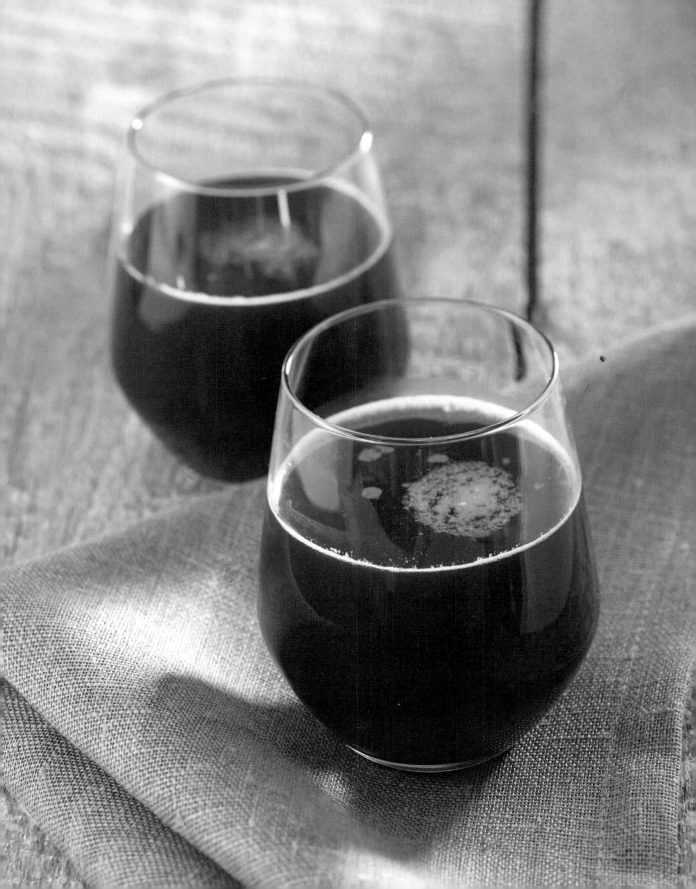

✦GLOW SMOOTHIE✦

This is the perfect smoothie for adding pep to your day. It also provides you with lasting nourishment so you can remain active for hours. Vanilla protein is not only sweet and scrumptious, it also provides easily digestible amino acids, which give you energy and protects the health of your organs and tissues. Avocado imparts a smooth and creamy texture as well as fiber to help you feel fuller longer. Spinach and kale deliver an abundance of phytochemicals that protect your heart and beautify your skin, and camu camu powder offers potent vitamin C for immunity. All of these nutrient powerhouses are blended with creamy and sweet banana, which keeps your body hydrated, a must when you are on the go.

Time: 5 minutes

Equipment: Blender

Yields: Approximately one 20-ounce (570 ml) smoothie

Ingredients:

3 tablespoons (23 g) vanilla plant protein powder (such as pea or hemp)

½ medium naval orange, peeled

½ medium banana

¼ medium avocado, peeled and pitted

1 small handful spinach

2 large kale leaves, de-ribbed and chopped

1 teaspoon camu camu powder

1 piece (½ inch, or 1 cm) fresh ginger, peeled

1½ cups (355 ml) unsweetened almond milk

Preparation:

In a blender, combine all the ingredients.

Blend on high for 20 seconds. Enjoy immediately and sip slowly.

✦LEMON TWIST SMOOTHIE✦

Luscious lemon, what a zany citrus fruit. When paired with sweet pomegranate, the result is a to die for medley of complementary flavors. This might as well be considered a vitamin C tonic since you are getting concentrated levels of the antioxidant from the lemon juice and zest and the camu camu powder. Pomegranate, also rich in vitamin C, protects against all kinds of cancers and is a powerful heart nourisher. Yacon syrup adds sweet balance to this tangy lemon twist, while also delivering digestion-enhancing nutrients.

Time: 10 minutes

Equipment: Blender

Yield: Approximately one 16-ounce (475 ml) smoothie

Ingredients:

1 medium lemon, juiced

⅛ teaspoon lemon zest

½ teaspoon camu camu powder

2 cups (475 ml) pomegranate juice (no sugar added variety)

2 tablespoons (13 g) yacon syrup

5 to 6 ice cubes

Preparation:

In a blender, combine all the ingredients.

Blend on high for 20 seconds or until smooth. Enjoy!

✦PINK LEMONADE✦

This is pink lemonade like you've never had before. Unlike the varieties found in restaurant soda dispensers, this blend is more tangy than sweet due to the natural sugars coming only from hydrating coconut water and fiber-rich raspberries. Goji juice provides a mega-burst of antioxidants and a mildly sweet and tangy flavor, and orange, lemon, and camu camu powder contribute sharp tartness and loads of vitamin C.

Time: 5 minutes

Equipment: Blender

Yield: Approximately one 16-ounce (475 ml) pink lemonade

Ingredients:

½ cup (120 ml) Pure Goji Juice (see page 12)

½ cup (118 ml) fresh-pressed orange juice

1 medium lemon, juiced

½ cup (125 g) frozen raspberries

½ cup (120 ml) coconut water

½ teaspoon camu camu powder

Preparation:

In a blender, combine all the ingredients.

Blend on high for 20 seconds. Enjoy immediately and sip slowly.

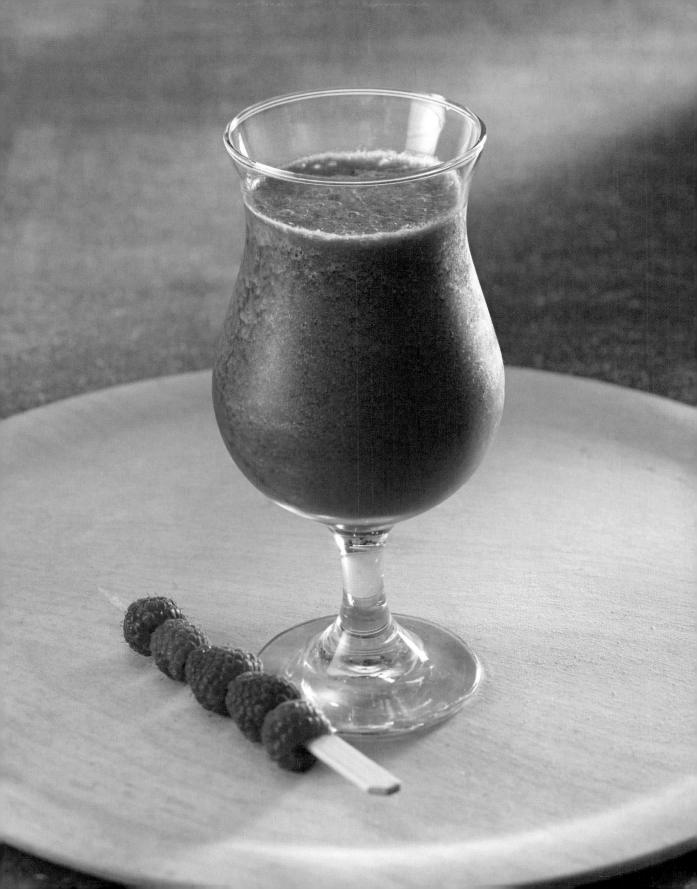

CHAPTER 3

MAQUI

DISEASE-FIGHTING ANTIOXIDANT

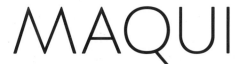

FEATURED RECIPES

Chilean Passion Juice

Maqui Magic Smoothie

Purple Haze Smoothie

Stone Fruit Smoothie

Antioxidant Berry Punch

South America is home to countless exotic fruits, all with incredible health properties. One that is as beautiful as it is nutritious is maqui, a small purple berry grown on shrubs in the Patagonia region of Chile. Its blackberry-like flavor is tangy and sweet, making it a commonly used fruit in Chilean wine blends. As a matter of fact, the berry is used so often in this capacity that maqui is also sometimes called Chilean wineberry. For more than five hundred years, the Mapuche Indians of South America have credited their health, strength, and stamina to their regular consumption of maqui. Let's take a look at why.

CHOLESTEROL-COMBATTING ANTIOXIDANT PROTECTION

Maqui contains a high concentration of anthocyanins, a potent antioxidant that gives the berry its vibrant purple hue. Other sources of the flavonoid include cherries, raspberries, blueberries, blackberries, currants, purple and red grapes, strawberries, and red wine. Anthocyanins provide multiple health benefits, including reducing oxidative stress as well as lowering blood pressure and bad cholesterol levels.

In a 2002 report published in the *Journal of Agricultural and Food Chemistry*, tests conducted on human cells that were treated with maqui extract showed a decrease in LDL ("bad") cholesterol levels. What's more, the antioxidants reduced oxidation of LDL cholesterol, meaning they neutralized damaging free radicals.

In addition, in the U.S. National Library of Medicine, a report was published in March 2010 in which three researchers from the Department of Nutritional Sciences at Oklahoma State University evaluated anthocyanins in clinical studies and noted they were associated with reduced cardiovascular risk.

OXIDATIVE STRESS PROTECTION

Oxidative stress is a burden placed on our bodies that comes by way of chemicals in the foods we eat, exposure to environmental toxins, as well as harmful lifestyle habits such as regularly drinking soda, smoking, using drugs, or lacking stress management or exercise. The greater the oxidative load, the greater the free radical proliferation.

In an article published in December 2004 in the *Journal of Biomedicine and Biotechnology*, two researchers, Wei Zhang and Izabela Konczak, described the effect anthocyanins have on human health. In the report, they stated that the antioxidant acts as an effective free radical scavenger, aiding in the neutralization of these harmful particles. Consumption of this group of antioxidants may play a significant role in the prevention of lifestyle-related diseases such as cancer, diabetes, and cardiovascular disease, they said.

MAQUI BERRIES BEAUTIFY

When we are burdened with oxidative stress, which all of us are, we are more prone to experience inflammation of our tissues, cells, and organs, the largest of which is our skin. During this process, connective tissues become damaged, thus leading to sallow, loose, or wrinkled skin. Anthocyanins boost collagen production, helping to firm and tone the skin and promote a more youthful texture and glow.

Sourcing and Care of Maqui

You will likely not come by fresh maqui berries outside of South America, so your best resource for this amazing fruit is freeze-dried powder. It is essential to look for brands that are 100 percent certified organic and produce powder with an opaque purple color. Powders that are light purple or that have a brown cast were overly processed and are thus void of nutrients. Look for freeze-dried powder online or at your natural food market. This convenient and versatile powder can be added to smoothies, juices, and desserts, sprinkled over hot cereal, or added to baked goods. Always store in your freezer or refrigerator to maintain freshness and use within four months of opening. According to raw maqui powder manufacturers, the suggested serving size is 2 teaspoons (5 g) of the powder daily. I suggest starting with one and working up from there.

✦CHILEAN PASSION JUICE✦

After one sip, you just might find yourself feeling passionate about introducing maqui into your diet. This juice tastes incredible! And the blend is bursting with vitamins, minerals, antioxidants, and enzymes. Pineapple is rich in bromelain, a potent digestive enzyme that aids in the breakdown of protein. Kale delivers sulfurous compounds that fight infection and detoxify the liver. Cucumber, a diuretic, aids in the elimination of toxins and carcinogens, and deliciously sweet and tangy maqui protects your heart and helps keep your cholesterol levels in check.

Time: 10 minutes

Equipment: Juicer

Yields: Approximately one 16-ounce (475 ml) juice

Ingredients:

4 medium kale leaves

1 medium cucumber, ends trimmed

¼ medium fresh pineapple, ends trimmed, skin cut away, and cut into spears

½ teaspoon maqui powder

Preparation:

Pass the kale, cucumber, and pineapple through a juicer in the order specified.

Transfer to a serving glass, stir in maqui powder, and enjoy!

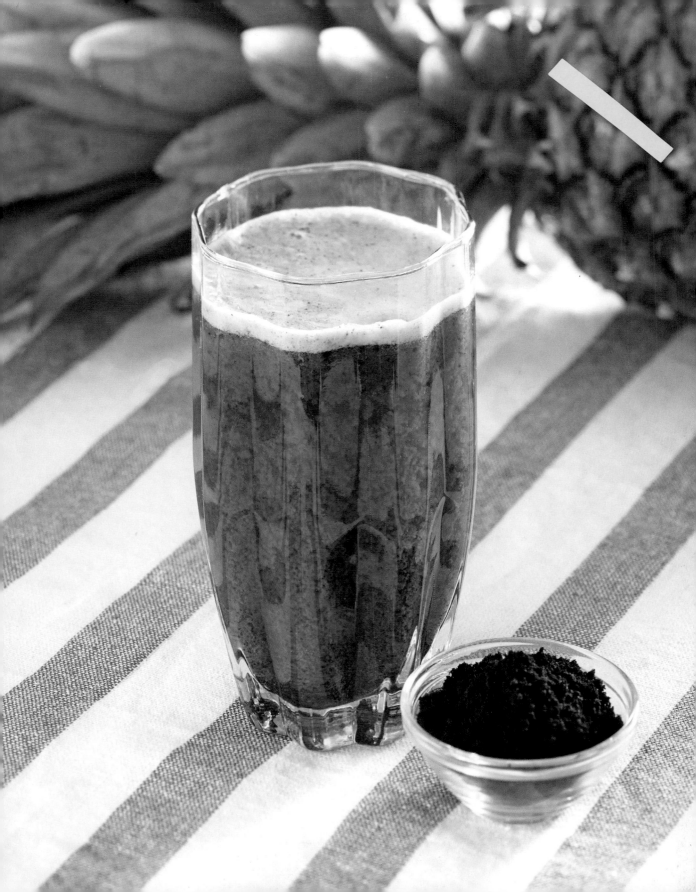

✦MAQUI MAGIC SMOOTHIE✦

This smoothie is oh so creamy and delicious it will make your mouth hum. The blend of rich and velvety cacao pairs magically with sweet and tangy maqui. You will get to indulge in decadent flavor while feeling nourished to the core. Raw cacao contains more than sixty antioxidants, and maqui is a leading source of anthocyanins, a heart-healthy phytonutrient. Watch out when these two notoriously nutritious superfoods come together. They are champions at protecting your heart, beautifying your body, and aiding in the elimination of nasty toxins you no longer want in your bod! Oh, and the flavor—think exotic and magical.

Time: 5 minutes

Equipment: Blender

Yield: Approximately one 20-ounce (570 ml) smoothie

Ingredients:

½ cup (75 g) fresh or frozen blueberries

1 tablespoon (6 g) raw cacao powder

1 cup (235 ml) coconut water

1 cup (235 ml) unsweetened almond milk

½ medium avocado, peeled and pitted

2 teaspoons (5 g) maqui powder

1 teaspoon vanilla extract

6 ice cubes

Preparation:

In a blender, combine all the ingredients.

Blend on high for 20 seconds. Enjoy immediately and sip slowly.

✦PURPLE HAZE SMOOTHIE✦

This luscious smoothie will take you away to the islands with the distinct tropical flavors of coconut and banana. Fresh orange juice adds zing and vibrancy to the sweet ingredients while delivering an abundance of vitamin C. This delicious shake keeps you hydrated due to the high potassium content of coconut water and banana. Unsweetened coconut is comprised of mostly medium-chain fatty acids. These chains of molecules are not as complex as the long-chain acids of most saturated fats, which makes them more easily assimilated. Because they break down and are assimilated faster in the body, they rev your metabolism. This sounds like a perfect blend to start the day, if you ask me!

Time: 5 minutes

Equipment: Blender

Yield: Approximately one 20-ounce (570 ml) smoothie

Ingredients:

1 small banana

2 tablespoons (10 g) unsweetened shredded coconut

2 teaspoons (5 g) maqui powder

1 cup (235 ml) coconut water

1 cup (235 ml) fresh squeezed orange juice

6 ice cubes

Preparation:

In a blender, combine all the ingredients.

Blend on high for 20 seconds. Enjoy!

✦STONE FRUIT SMOOTHIE✦

Summer is stone fruit season, and the family includes apricots, cherries, peaches, nectarines, and plums. A simple and delicious way to utilize some favorites is in this remarkably delicious smoothie. Nectarines are rich in vitamin C, which makes skin glow and increases elasticity for better tone. Cherries are full of antioxidants that protect the heart and ensure healthy cholesterol levels. The addition of walnuts provides omega-3 fatty acids that boost brain health, and avocado supports hormone regulation and healthy digestion. It's not too shabby of a nutrient lineup for such a creamy, sweet, and scrumptious treat!

Time: 10 minutes

Equipment: Blender

Yield: Approximately one 20-ounce (570 ml) smoothie

Ingredients:

½ medium fresh nectarine, stone removed and chopped, or ½ cup (125 g) frozen peaches or nectarine slices

½ plum, stone removed

¼ medium avocado, peeled and pitted

6 pitted cherries

2 pitted medjool dates

1 cup (235 ml) unsweetened almond milk

2 tablespoons (28 ml) water

1 tablespoon (8 g) walnuts

½ teaspoon vanilla extract

Pinch sea salt

¼ teaspoon maqui powder

Preparation:

In a blender, combine all the ingredients except the maqui powder.

Blend on high for 20 seconds.

Pour into a serving glass, sprinkle with maqui powder, and enjoy!

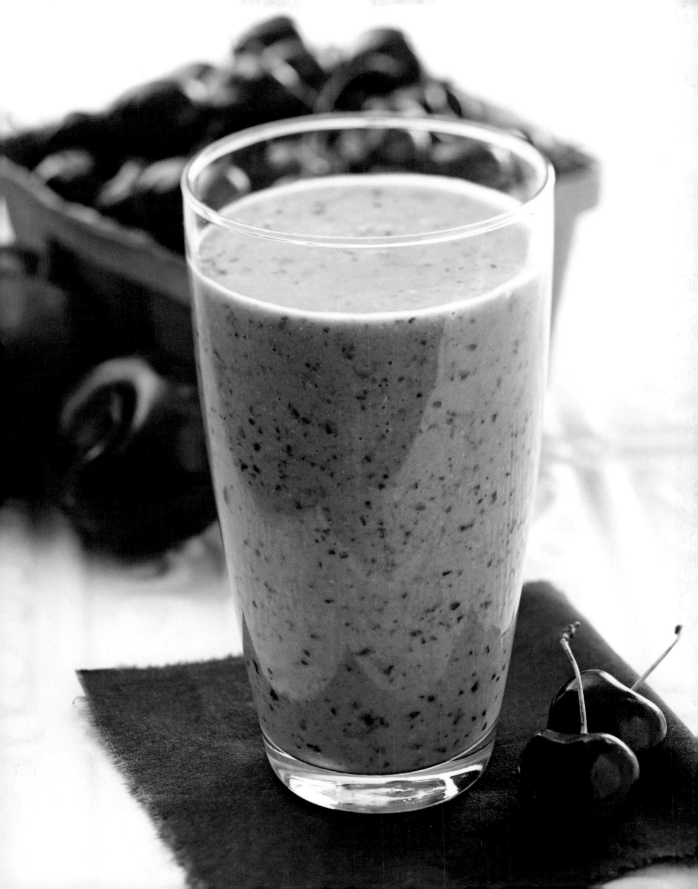

✦ANTIOXIDANT BERRY✦ PUNCH

Throw a party and wow your guests with this nutritious, nonalcoholic punch that is sure to turn them into raving juice fans. A fresh-pressed blend of sweet apple, detoxifying cucumber and parsley, and digestion-enhancing red grapes create the base for this festive tonic. Add some sparkling mineral water, stir in heart-healthy maqui powder and antioxidant-bursting berries, and you are ready for entertaining!

Time: 15 minutes

Equipment: Juicer and large pitcher

Yield: Approximately ten ¾ cup (175 ml) servings

Ingredients:

1 large handful parsley

1 pound red seedless grapes, room temperature

3 medium cucumbers, ends trimmed

4 medium semisweet apples (such as Fuji or Gala), halved

1 tablespoon (8 g) maqui powder

2 cups (475 ml) sparkling mineral water

2 cups (290 g) mixed berries (fresh or frozen and any variety you choose)

Fresh mint leaves for garnish

Preparation:

Pass the parsley, grapes, cucumbers, and apples through a juicer in the order specified.

Transfer to a pitcher, stir in the maqui powder, mineral water, berries, and mint leaves. Serve chilled.

LUCUMA

THE "GOLD OF THE INCAS"

FEATURED RECIPES

Post-Workout Revival Smoothie

Creamy Carrot Crush Juice

Salted Caramel Smoothie

Buttery Banana Smoothie

Anytime Nog

Which South American fruit has rough green skin with creamy flesh and a large pit in the center? If this description strikes up the image of the beloved Californian favorite, the avocado, then we need to brush up on our exotic fruits! This one is a national favorite in its homeland of Peru and is often used for its seductively sweet maple flavor in South American ice creams. Lucuma is one fruit worth knowing about, and you'll soon see why. The whole fruit is very difficult to come by in the states, but you may find the frozen pulp in Hispanic markets. Additionally, the commonly dried and ground powder is available through natural food distributers in the United States and around the globe. This convenient form allows for it to be used in a variety of ways.

A LOOK AT LUCUMA

Similar in shape, color, and size to a large avocado, the lucuma is filled with a sweet, rosy-hued yellow flesh. It is often called eggfruit for the traits it shares with its cousin the canistel. Both have a slightly creamy flesh that resembles cooked egg yolk. Lucuma is very nutritious, having high levels of carotene, vitamin B3, and other B vitamins, thus it plays an important role in bone and protein formation, healthy digestion, and hormone balance.

Lucuma was considered a revered symbol of fertility and life to the inhabitants of ancient Peru. They believed the fruit embodied mystical powers and both respected and feared it but also depended on it for its curative and medicinal properties.

Lucuma powder is derived from the fruit's dried flesh and can be incorporated into a wide variety of foods. Lucuma is most often described as having a mellow, maple-vanilla flavor, or a flavor similar to that of caramel mixed with sweet potato. Like most fruits, the flavor can change a bit throughout the seasons and from year to year.

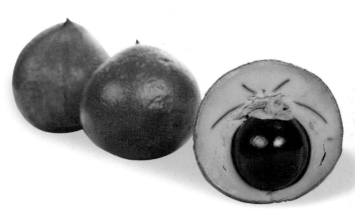

COMPLEX CARBS EQUAL NATURAL NUTRITION

In addition to containing carotene and B vitamins, lucuma also boasts high levels of immune-supporting antioxidants. It is also high in fiber and essential minerals such as iron. In addition, lucuma is lower in sugar content when compared to other tropical fruits such as mangoes, bananas, and pineapples, producing less of a caloric or glycemic burden. Instead, lucuma's complex carbohydrates are slowly absorbed over a long period of time, causing only a minimal rise in blood sugar levels. Complex carbohydrates are also important for their roles in aiding mineral absorption and the formation of fatty acids. Fatty acids are essential nutrients, meaning we do not manufacture them on our own and must absorb them from the foods we eat. These essential nutrients such as omega-3 support the health of our brain and heart.

AN ALL-INCLUSIVE CULINARY CONTRIBUTOR

Lucuma powder makes a tantalizing, healthy addition to your diet. One of its trademark benefits is that it blends seamlessly into so many different foods and enhances a variety of flavors. You might want to try lucuma as a nutritious addition to gluten-free flour blends to use in recipes for muffins, cookies, pancakes, and even birthday cakes! I also recommend replacing high-glycemic sweeteners (white sugar, beet sugar, cane sugar, high fructose corn syrup, and agave) with lucuma powder in sweets drinks, desserts, cereals, and baked goods.

If you are a do-it-yourself raw or vegan food aficionado and are just beginning to experiment with making sweet treats at home, there are endless ways

Sourcing and Care of Lucuma

Many popular health food chains as well as your local natural food market may carry packaged lucuma powder. However, if your local market doesn't currently stock this amazing superfood, you may purchase it online through popular websites that sell food supplements or superfood products. Lucuma powder should appear as a loose powder that ranges in color from off-white to rosy beige.

Lucuma powder is best stored in an airtight glass container out of direct sunlight. To prevent exposure to moisture, which will cause clumping and rancidity, it is best stored in its original bag or in a well-sealed glass jar in a cabinet. Properly stored, lucuma will remain nutritionally potent for up to a year.

to fit lucuma into the mix. For example, I am a huge fan of making raw superfood chocolates, and lucuma is my superstar ingredient for adding a creamy milk chocolate texture and flavor to soothe the mild bitterness of raw cacao. Try lucuma in raw ice cream, hot chocolate, chia porridge, dressings, sauces, and smoothies, such as the ones I've dreamed up in the following pages.

Superfoods that blend well with lucuma are raw cacao, maca, sacha inchi, hemp seeds, bee pollen, and chia, all of which are in this book!

✦POST-WORKOUT REVIVAL✦ SMOOTHIE

Get your healthy dose of sweet, mapley lucuma powder with this super-powered wonder smoothie! This fruity, slightly frozen fiesta of flavor is pumped up with enzymes and electrolytes. Mildly creamy with tropical overtones, this is one of my favorite post-workout drinks because it supplies my body with complex carbs, protein, electrolytes, and plenty of vitamins and phytonutrients. Of course, you don't have to wait until after working out to prepare this beauty. It's the perfect meal replacement shake and is a great way to sneak some extra protein into kids with picky eating habits. After all, few children can resist a creamy, sweet fruit treat.

Time: 5 minutes

Equipment: Blender

Yield: Approximately one 20-ounce (570 ml) smoothie

Ingredients:
½ cup (90 g) frozen mango chunks

¼ cup (40 g) frozen pineapple pieces

1½ cups (355 ml) coconut water

½ medium banana

2 tablespoons (15 g) vanilla plant protein powder (such as pea or hemp)

2 tablespoons (30 g) lucuma powder

Preparation:

In a blender, combine all the ingredients.

Blend on high for 20 seconds until smooth. Share and enjoy!

+CREAMY CARROT+ CRUSH JUICE

If you are looking for a way to cover your As and bump up your Bs, this is one juicy jubilee you've got to try! This is truly an excellent way to get a healthy dose of these vitamins. Carrots are high in carotenoids, which the body uses to synthesize vitamin A. It is a rare treat when you find a juice as silky and scrumptious as this one. Creamy, soothing almond milk and luscious lucuma take our sweet friend carrot juice to the next level. Enter this one into your repertoire as a family favorite because it's sure to become one.

Time: 10 minutes

Equipment: Juicer and blender

Yield: Approximately one 16-ounce (475 ml) juice

Ingredients:
6 medium carrots
1 cup (235 ml) unsweetened
    almond milk
1 tablespoon (15 g) lucuma powder

Preparation:
Pass the carrots through a juicer.

Transfer to a blender and combine with the almond milk and lucuma powder. Blend on high for 20 seconds until a smooth consistency is achieved. Savor every sip!

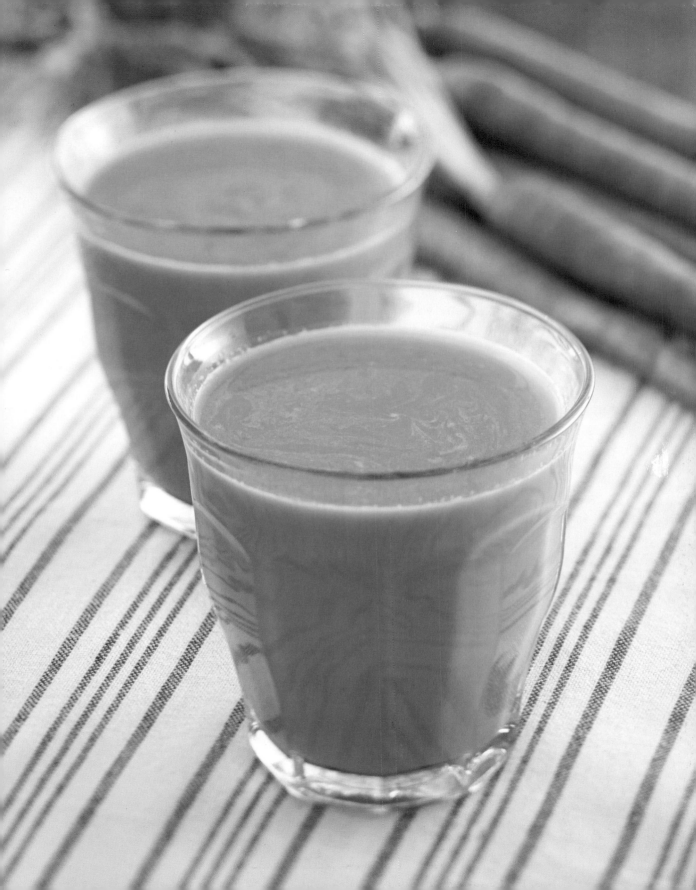

✦SALTED CARAMEL✦ SMOOTHIE

One of my all-time favorite flavors is caramel! I love its natural fusion of maple and sugar and its sweet, syrupy consistency. Traditional caramel is derived from browned sugar and dairy milk, but you'll be amazed by how similar in flavor a combination of lucuma powder and fresh dates can be. This smoothie is utterly sensual. It's an absolute treat after dinner or a wonderfully healthy way to trick your kids into having a healthy breakfast. It also makes the most amazing ice cream. Just throw the entire smoothie recipe into your ice cream maker and follow the manufacturer's directions or freeze in ice cube trays and push them through a masticating juicer. Either way, you'll end up with a bowl full of creamy decadence no one would ever suspect to be dairy-free!

Time: 10 minutes

Equipment: Blender

Yield: Approximately one 20-ounce (570 ml) smoothie

Ingredients:

2 tablespoons (15 g) vanilla plant protein powder (such as pea or hemp)

2 tablespoons (30 g) lucuma powder

¼ teaspoon sea salt

1 teaspoon vanilla extract

¼ cup (35 g) cashews

2 cups (475 ml) unsweetened almond milk

5 pitted medjool dates

Preparation:

In a blender, combine all the ingredients.

Blend on high for about thirty seconds. Enjoy!

✦BUTTERY BANANA✦ SMOOTHIE

Sometimes you just need something decadently sweet, smooth, and silky to soothe away the hard edges of the day. This calcium-rich smoothie is dangerously addicting. Its milkshake-like taste is a sweet treat on days when you can't escape the heat, and it is the smoothie you want for a late afternoon pick-me-up. The complex carbs and excellent mineral content provide slow-release energy for hours on end. This Buttery Banana Smoothie also has nourishing and lasting power from loads of protein and fiber, making it a great way to start the day. You can even throw in a handful of spinach to pump up the nutrient content and give it a monstrous green twist kids love! Just don't tell them why it's green.

Time: 5 minutes

Equipment: Blender

Yield: Approximately one 24-ounce (700 ml) smoothie

Ingredients:
3 tablespoons (48 g) almond butter
2 tablespoons (30 g) lucuma powder
2 cups (475 ml) unsweetened
    almond milk
1 medium frozen banana
3 pitted medjool dates
¼ teaspoon sea salt
6 ice cubes

Preparation:
In a blender, combine all the ingredients.

Blend on high for 20 seconds. Serve and enjoy!

✦ANYTIME NOG✦

Most people think of nog as a drink reserved for the winter holidays. I beg to differ! This exotically scented concoction inspires those warm, fuzzy feelings through any season and for any reason. Warm, spicy nutmeg is mildly mood enhancing and pleasantly nostalgic. I love to drink this nog alongside my morning chia seed porridge or even as an afternoon snack. It instantly transports me to those places where my warmest, coziest memories reside.

Time: 5 minutes

Equipment: Blender

Yield: Approximately one 12-ounce (355 ml) nog

Ingredients:
1¼ cups (285 ml) unsweet-
  ened almond milk
2 tablespoons (30 g) lucuma powder
½ teaspoon vanilla extract
¼ teaspoon ground nutmeg
2 tablespoons (15 g) hemp seeds
2 tablespoons (40 g) maple syrup
⅛ teaspoon sea salt

Preparation:
In a blender, combine all the ingredients.

Blend on high for 20 seconds. Serve with a sprinkle of nutmeg and enjoy the moment!

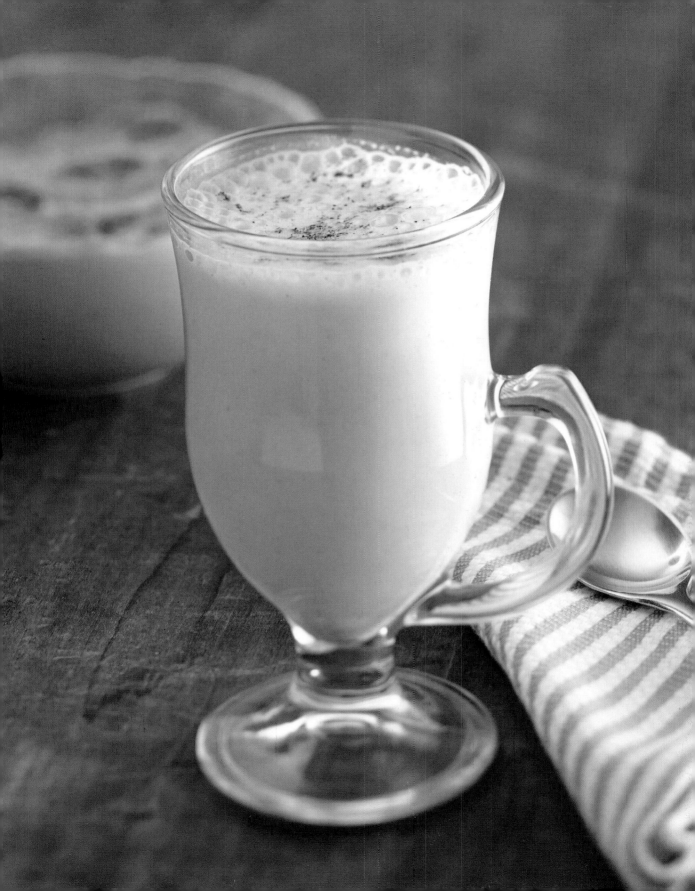

CHAPTER 5

GOLDEN BERRIES

PROTEIN-PACKED POWERHOUSES

FEATURED RECIPES

Andes Sunrise Smoothie

Cape Berry Squeeze Juice

Caramel Cream Pop Smoothie

Golden Ticket Juice

Orange Cream Smoothie

How many years have you been noshing on dried cranberries? Probably for as long as you can remember, right? I am sure you have been adding them to salads, sprinkling them on your breakfast cereal, or tossing them into your favorite trail mix. But aren't you a tad burned out on these little guys? Yes, they may be convenient and antioxidant-rich, but there's room for another berry, one that has been around for thousands of years, growing in the tropics of three continents, and hailed as a remarkable super fruit. Even its name is powerful and commanding. It is the golden berry.

You may not recognize the name because this fruit is known by other names, depending on the region in which it is cultivated. Those from the Cape of South Africa are referred to as Cape gooseberries, and when harvested in South America, they take the name Incan berry.

Prior to being dried, these small golden fruits resemble small yellow tomatos or cherries. The delicate berry is shrouded in an aesthetically pleasing lantern-shaped paper husk and protected by fleshy pulp. You would think by its texture and shape that the golden berry is a relative of the cherry, but the super fruit is more closely related to the tomatillo.

Once sun dried, the berry is plump like a raisin, golden in color, and rich with seeds, a characteristic of its tomatillo relative. The flavor profile of the golden berry is distinct, with a robust citrus tang and a sweet finish, making it ideal for jams, chutneys, and salsas; tossing with green and grain salads; and including in your favorite juices and smoothies.

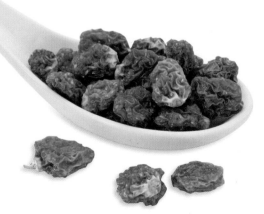

THRONE-WORTHY
HEALTH BENEFITS

This revered berry deserves royal praise for its health benefits. In a comprehensive study published in February 2010, researchers determined that the phyto-compound 4β-hydroxywithanolide, found in golden berries, inhibits the growth of existing lung cancer cells.

In addition, the golden berry is an excellent source of vitamin A. Adequate intake of this fat-soluble vitamin is critical for the health of your eyes and skin. It is also a powerful antioxidant and supports the neutralization of free radical activity in the body. You can receive 50 percent of your daily required amount (800 mcg) in just ¼ cup (30 g) of golden berries. The super berries are also composed of 5 percent pectin, a soluble fiber that supports healthy gut function and bowel regularity.

This tiny little fruit is composed of 16 percent protein and contains vitamins B1, B2, B6, and B12, needed for hundreds of bodily functions including stress reduction, energy production, metabolism, tissue repair, heart protection, and hormone regulation. Guess what else? The golden fruit is also abundant in phosphorous, a highly absorbable and vital mineral that aids in strengthening and building bone and tissue.

Enjoy the berries by the handful to get the full spectrum of their sweetness and tang. You can also blend them into smoothies, add them to your cereals and salads, or include them in stews. If you wish to get really creative, experiment with highly concentrated golden berry powder, found online or in natural food stores. I like to make smoothies and then finish them with a sprinkling of berry dust for a vibrant garnish. The powder is also excellent for incorporating into desserts such as coconut ice cream or those where you might otherwise use a tangy fruit such as orange or grapefruit.

Sourcing and Care of Golden Berries

Unlike a lot of super fruits, golden berries are grown throughout the year. They flourish in South American and African regions as well as in the warm climates of Australia and Hawaii. A single plant can yield three hundred berries! The plant also matures quickly, making the fruit plentiful year-round. This is good news for you since the more abundant the fruit, the less it costs. The average price for dried berries in bulk is forty-five cents for a 2-tablespoon (15 g) serving. Buy in bulk and stock your pantry with the sun dried fruit. Store in airtight glass for up to six months.

+ANDES SUNRISE+ SMOOTHIE

Pineapple is not only a sweet and succulent fruit, it is also an effective digestive aid. The enzyme bromelain supports protein assimilation and has anti-inflammatory properties. Coconut water and cilantro are cooling to the body and refreshing. The two marry nicely with sweet pineapple, tangy golden berry, and tart lime in this tantalizing tropical delight.

Time: 5 minutes

Equipment: Blender

Yield: Approximately one 20-ounce (570 ml) smoothie

Ingredients:
½ cup (85 g) frozen or
   fresh pineapple

1 tablespoon (15 ml) fresh lime juice

2 tablespoons (15 g) dried
   golden berries

1 small handful cilantro leaves

¾ cup (175 ml) coconut water

½ cup (120 ml) coconut milk

½ teaspoon vanilla extract

Preparation:
In a blender, combine all the ingredients.

Blend until smooth. Enjoy immediately and sip slowly.

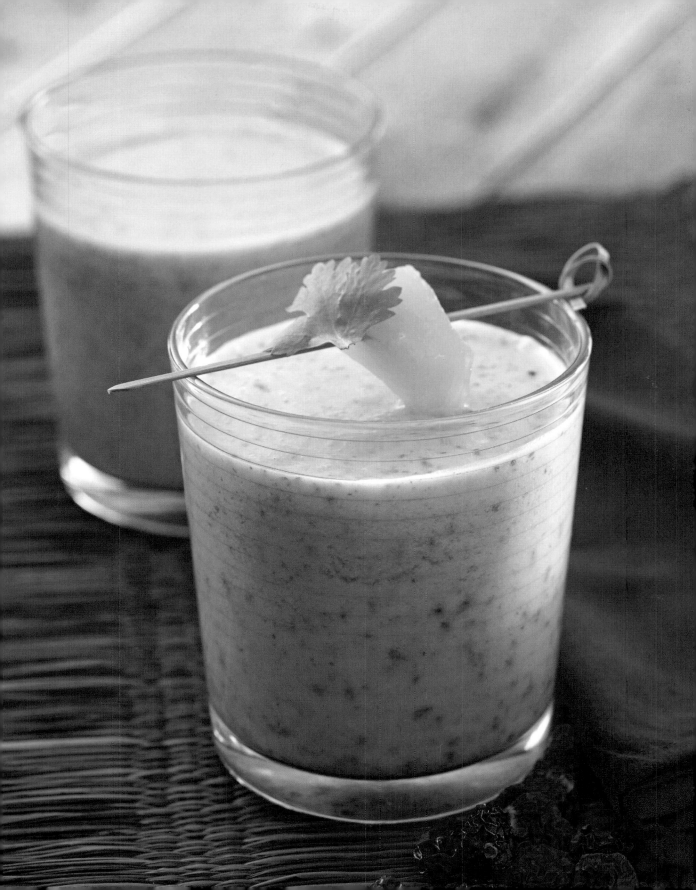

✦CAPE BERRY SQUEEZE✦ JUICE

Winter months bring colds and flu, but kiwi delivers relief in the form of immune-boosting properties such as vitamin C. Kiwi contains more of this essential vitamin than a medium-sized orange. It also imparts a sweet and tangy flavor that pairs beautifully with hydrating coconut water and fresh cucumber. A touch of golden berry powder boosts the antioxidant content of this fresh juice and adds a tart finish.

Time: 5 minutes

Equipment: Juicer and large glass jar

Yield: Approximately one 16-ounce (475 ml) juice

Ingredients:
2 medium cucumbers
3 kiwi, skin cut away
¼ cup (60 ml) coconut water
½ teaspoon golden berry powder

Preparation:
Pass the cucumber and kiwi through a juicer.

Transfer to a large glass jar and stir in the coconut water and golden berry powder. Enjoy immediately and sip slowly.

✦CARAMEL CREAM POP✦ SMOOTHIE

Whenever you crave a sugary treat, reach for this low-glycemic, luscious smoothie. The inclusion of lucuma, a super fruit with a rich maple and caramel taste, delivers sweetness without spiking your blood sugar levels. This makes an excellent workout recovery drink with the inclusion of protein powder and potassium-rich banana. You will also benefit from an abundance of golden berry's B vitamins as they reenergize you after activity.

Time: 5 minutes

Equipment: Blender

Yield: Approximately one 20-ounce (570 ml) smoothie

Ingredients:
½ medium banana

1 teaspoon golden berry powder

2 tablespoons (15 g) vanilla plant protein powder (such as pea or hemp)

2 tablespoons (30 g) lucuma powder

1 teaspoon vanilla extract

1 cup (235 ml) unsweetened vanilla almond milk

5 to 6 ice cubes

Preparation:
In a blender, combine all the ingredients.

Blend until smooth. Enjoy immediately and sip slowly.

✦GOLDEN TICKET JUICE✦

This truly is a golden juice with its proliferation of nutrients and sweet and tangy taste. It is golden in color due to golden berry powder, yellow beets, and vibrant orange carrots. The beets oxygenate and detoxify your blood, carrots beautify your skin and protect your eyes with their abundance of vitamins A and E, and apples deliver gut-friendly bacteria and provide a sweet balance to the subtle tang of protein-rich golden berry powder.

Time: 5 minutes

Equipment: Juicer

Yield: Approximately one 16-ounce (475 ml) juice

Ingredients:

1 medium golden beet, ends trimmed

4 large carrots, ends trimmed

1½ sweet apples (such as Red Delicious), quartered

1 medium lemon, peeled, with pith intact

1 teaspoon golden berry powder

Preparation:

Pass the golden beet, carrots, apples, and lemon through a juicer.

Transfer to a serving glass and sprinkle with golden berry powder. Enjoy immediately and sip slowly.

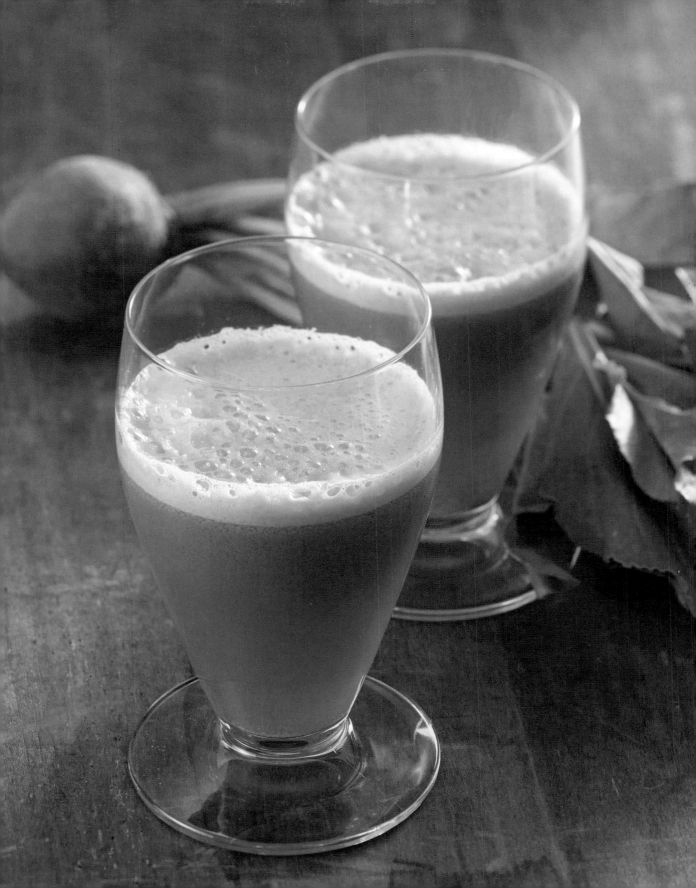

✦ORANGE CREAM✦ SMOOTHIE

Reminiscent of a frozen orange cream pop but made with nourishing ingredients, this smoothie blends the scrumptious and complementary flavors of vanilla and sweet orange. The juicy citrus fruit boosts your immune system, and the tang of this smoothie is balanced with fiber-rich and naturally sweet dates. Coconut milk and oil not only stave off hunger with their friendly fat content, they are also responsible for giving this smoothie its rich and creamy texture. The addition of vanilla plant protein powder delivers the distinct and delectable Creamsicle flavor while helping you feel deeply nourished.

Time: 5 minutes

Equipment: Blender

Yield: Approximately one 20-ounce (570 ml) smoothie

Ingredients:

2 medium navel oranges, peeled

2 tablespoons (15 g) dried golden berries

3 pitted medjool dates

1 cup (235 ml) coconut milk

2 tablespoons (15 g) vanilla plant protein powder (such as pea or hemp)

1 tablespoon (14 g) coconut oil

Preparation:

In a blender, combine all the ingredients.

Blend on high for 20 seconds or until smooth. Enjoy immediately and sip slowly.

CACAO

MAGNESIUM WONDER FRUIT

FEATURED RECIPES
CB&J Smoothie
Hidden Greens Smoothie
Chocolate-Dunked Monkey Smoothie
Mexi-Choco Froth
Chocolate Ginger Orange Twist Smoothie

Cocoa . . . cacao . . . chocolate . . . chocolat . . .
I might as well just say pure decadence. The rich
and tantalizing flavor of unadulterated cacao has
invoked feelings of pleasure for centuries. Despite
the universal satisfaction achieved with chocolate
indulgence, the varieties responsible for the elation
are not created equal. There is a significant difference
between commercially produced chocolate and minimally processed, dark variations, and it is important
to understand the distinctions.

Let's begin with the difference between cacao and
cocoa. Cacao originates from the Theobroma cacao,
a tree native to South America that produces seeds
used to make cocoa. There are many theories as to
where the term "cocoa" emerged. According to the
June 2008 issue of *Positive Health* magazine, in
1828, a Dutch chocolatier invented a machine
that extracted and separated the cacao butter
from roasted cacao beans and their liquor. The
process also treated the chocolate with alkalinizing
agents such as baking soda to neutralize acidity,

a process called dutching. The chocolatier's invention
then pressed the beans' resulting paste into blocks,
which were later ground into powder for baked goods
and drinks. He called the resulting and versatile
commercially produced product cocoa. The name and
processed product became globally accepted, and
"cacao," until recently, became a term of the past.

The reintroduction of the word "cacao" to our
modern vernacular has quite a bit to do with the raw
food movement. Raw pioneers such as David Wolfe
are forever on a quest to discover foods grown in
nature with the greatest saturation of nutrients. In
search of these life-affirming superfoods, these raw
foodists found themselves back at cacao, the actual
bean grown abundantly in South America. During
their journey, they discovered the many ways this

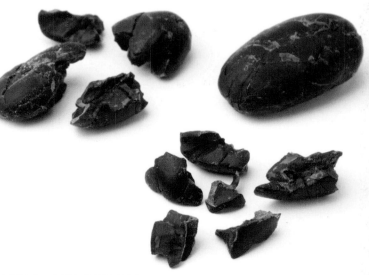

Sourcing and Care of Cacao

Cacao can be used in many ways. For instance, cacao butter can be purchased in blocks or jars and is excellent for making raw chocolate truffles and as a binder for energy bars. It also serves as a luxurious skin moisturizer! Cacao powder can be blended into smoothies, puddings, and ice creams or used in baked goods. It also adds unique flavor and dimension to Mexican, Southwestern, and Spanish dishes such as mole and chili. Cacao nibs are a healthy and delicious snack eaten piece by piece. They also add crunch and a notable element of bitterness to sweet smoothies and trail mix.

When purchasing cacao, look for products that are minimally processed with at least 70 percent cacao. Also be sure treats are made with natural sweeteners and without emulsifiers like soy lecithin.

Because of the high fat content of pure cacao, to prevent rancidity store in airtight glass and in a cool and dry environment such as your pantry. Alternatively, you may store cacao products in your refrigerator. Powder and butter will remain fresh if stored this way for up to one year, and bars maintain their taste for up to three months.

incredible fruit supports longevity. Suppliers of raw food products began cultivating, harvesting, and distributing a variety of raw cacao ingredients and so the word cacao was restored to our vocabulary.

Interest in cacao and its health benefits has made its way into the mainstream. Raw cacao powder and butter and dark chocolate bars and treats are readily available and are being infused with ingredients such as goji berries, ginger, orange, chili pepper, sea salt, and even lavender.

WAIST SLIMMING DECADENCE

The main difference between beneficial and commercially produced cacao products is that the latter are full of junk. Artificial ingredients such as high fructose corn syrup, refined sugars, dairy solids, and emulsifiers such as soy lecithin are responsible for chocolate's bad reputation for promoting weight gain, increasing diabetes risk, and contributing to high cholesterol. It is the artificial ingredients, not the cacao, that have negative health implications. This is why health experts such as Andrew Weil, MD, Mark Hyman, MD, and Mehmet Oz, MD, suggest we eat only raw and dark chocolate products containing 70 percent or more cacao. Weil has said with cacao content that high, the presence of sugar is invariably lower. Minimally processed dark chocolate contains stearic acid, a saturated fat that does not raise LDL, or bad, cholesterol, he says, and he recommends enjoying an ounce or two (28 to 55 g) several times each week.

In 2011, an article written for AARP summarized research conducted at Harvard Medical School. Studies demonstrated how chocolate could reduce diabetes risk and support heart health. The comprehensive research included twenty-four chocolate studies involving 1,106 participants. Results showed that dark chocolate with at least 50 to 70 percent cacao lowered blood pressure in all participants. Study co-author Eric Ding, PhD, a clinical nutritionist and epidemiologist, said they also found cacao increases insulin sensitivity, which lowers the risk of diabetes. This is great news for chocoholics, as are claims that chocolate can aid in weight loss.

Research conducted by Hiroshige Itakura, MD, a Japanese physician at Ibaraki Christian University, suggests eating dark chocolate supports weight loss so long as the chocolate consumed is 70 percent cacao or more. It is also effective in weight reduction if the amount enjoyed is limited to fewer than 2 ounces (55 g) per day. He says the reasons for this are that cacao contains a polyphenol that assists in the absorption of glucose and burns fat, and theobromine, an alkaloid that contains serotonin reuptake inhibitors and gives chocolate its bitter flavor and reduces stress. When we are less stressed, we tend not to overeat and can more easily maintain or lose weight.

MAGNESIUM MAVEN

Cacao is one of the highest known whole food sources of magnesium. This essential mineral participates in more than three hundred bodily functions, yet is the mineral we are commonly deficient in. Often, we lack magnesium because of our food being grown in mineral-depleted soil or from not eating enough magnesium-rich foods. In addition, our absorption can be compromised because of constant exposure to environmental toxins, stress, food additives, preservatives, and stimulants such as caffeine.

Some of the tangible ways magnesium supports us is by improving bowel regularity. It also relaxes muscles, including your heart, so you feel a greater sense of calm. Common side effects of a magnesium deficiency include insomnia, headaches, muscle fatigue, cramps, soreness, constipation, and anxiety. A minimum of 300 mg of magnesium per day is the recommended adult daily allowance, and you get half that amount in just 2 tablespoons (12 g) of cacao powder or 1 ounce (28 g) of dark chocolate containing at least 70 percent cacao!

✦CB&J SMOOTHIE✦

A reinvention of the legendary peanut butter and jelly combo, this rich smoothie will have you reminiscing about your childhood. Raspberries, rich in antioxidants and fiber, pair magnificently with raw cacao butter and powder. You will feel deeply sated for hours from the abundance of heart-healthy fat found in the cacao ingredients as well as in the flax, which also contains an abundance of fiber. What's more? You will meet your daily magnesium requirement in just one serving of this scrumptious smoothie. Enjoy this nutrient-rich shake anytime and feel free to substitute strawberries, blackberries, or cherries for the raspberries if they are hard to come by.

Time: 5 minutes

Equipment: Blender

Yield: Approximately one 20-ounce (570 ml) smoothie

Ingredients:

1 cup (125 g) frozen or
    fresh raspberries

1 tablespoon (13 g) cacao butter

2 teaspoons (6 g) flax meal

1½ cups (355 ml) unsweet-
    ened almond milk

1 tablespoon (8 g) raw cacao powder

2 tablespoons (40 g) maple syrup

Pinch sea salt

5 to 6 ice cubes

Preparation:

In a blender, combine all the ingredients.

Blend on high for 20 seconds or until smooth. Enjoy immediately and sip slowly.

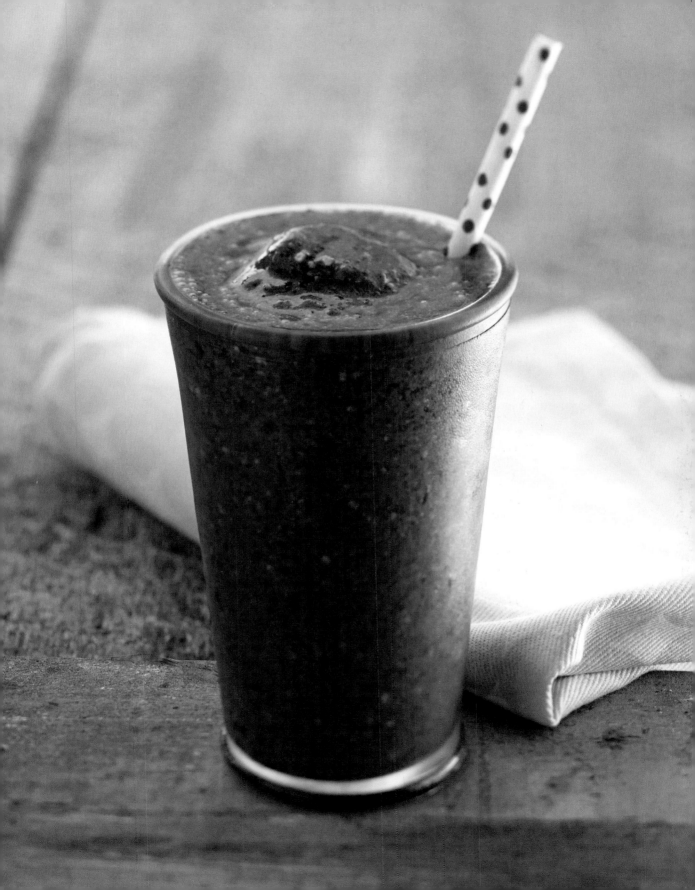

✦HIDDEN GREENS✦ SMOOTHIE

Get an entire day's worth of greens in one serving of this velvety dark chocolate smoothie. The cacao flavor is so pronounced that the abundance of broccoli, spinach, and kale nearly go undetected. The addition of maple syrup gently sweetens this creamy delight, and dates help to satisfy your hunger because of their high content of insoluble fiber. If you have children, start their day with this chocolate shake. They will never know just how healthy a treat they are getting!

Time: 5 minutes

Equipment: Blender

Yield: Approximately one 20-ounce (570 ml) smoothie

Ingredients:
2 large kale leaves, de-ribbed and chopped

2 large handfuls spinach

3 broccoli florets

3 pitted medjool dates

2 tablespoons (12 g) raw cacao powder

1½ cups (355 ml) unsweetened almond milk

2 tablespoons (40 g) maple syrup

5 to 6 ice cubes

Preparation:
In a blender, combine all the ingredients.

Blend on high for 20 seconds or until smooth. Enjoy immediately and sip slowly.

✦CHOCOLATE-DUNKED✦ MONKEY SMOOTHIE

The child in you will crave this chocolaty banana treat, and your heart will thank you for the cardiovascular-friendly alkaloids in the cacao. This smoothie contains a serving of plant-based protein, which helps you feel fuller longer, making it an excellent meal replacement. Banana provides potassium, which supports the balance of hydration, and fresh dates not only boost the smoothie's sweetness, they are also rich in fiber. Hidden beneath all of these yummy ingredients are two cups (60 g) of fresh spinach, giving you three servings of greens with cancer-fighting flavonoids.

Time: 5 minutes

Equipment: Blender

Yield: Approximately one 20-ounce (570 ml) smoothie

Ingredients:

1 medium banana

2 cups (60 g) spinach leaves

3 pitted medjool dates

2 tablespoons (12 g) raw cacao powder

2 tablespoons (15 g) chocolate plant protein powder (such as pea or hemp)

1½ cups (355 ml) unsweetened almond milk

5 to 6 ice cubes

Preparation:

In a blender, combine all the ingredients.

Blend on high for 20 seconds or until smooth. Enjoy immediately and sip slowly.

✦MEXI-CHOCO FROTH✦

An icy and frothy drink is ultra-refreshing, and this one is especially delicious with its Mexican flare. Magnesium-rich cacao is paired with anti-inflammatory cayenne, cinnamon, and clove for a taste that is decadently smoky, sweet, and spicy.

Time: 5 minutes

Equipment: Blender

Yield: Approximately one 12-ounce (355 ml) froth

Ingredients:

1 tablespoon (6 g) raw cacao powder

¼ teaspoon ground cinnamon

1/16 teaspoon ground cloves

1/16 teaspoon ground cayenne pepper

1/16 teaspoon ground nutmeg

1¼ cups (285 ml) unsweet-ened almond milk

2 tablespoons (40 g) maple syrup

10 ice cubes

Pinch sea salt

Preparation:

In a blender, combine all ingredients.

Blend on high until the ice is crushed and a slushy texture is achieved. Enjoy immediately and savor every frothy sip.

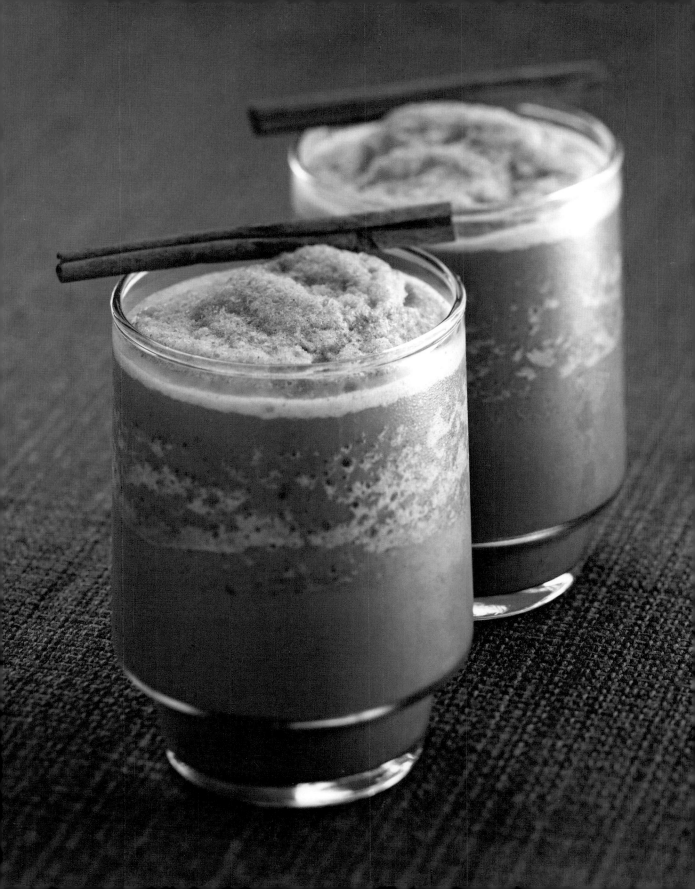

✦CHOCOLATE GINGER✦ ORANGE TWIST SMOOTHIE

Imagine indulging in a chocolate bar infused with ginger and succulent orange. Is your mouth watering yet? Enjoy these three distinct and scrumptious flavors in a treat you can sip anytime. Ginger has anti-inflammatory and immune-boosting properties; orange is rich in vitamin C; and avocado contains heart-healthy fat and fiber, which helps you feel full for hours. Raw cacao provides more than sixty-one antioxidants, so you don't have to feel guilty about having chocolate for breakfast.

Time: 5 minutes

Equipment: Blender

Yield: Approximately one 20-ounce (570 ml) smoothie

Ingredients:

2 tablespoons (12 g) raw cacao powder

1 tablespoon (13 g) cacao butter

¼ medium avocado, peeled and pitted

1 piece (½ inch, or 1 cm) fresh ginger, peeled

½ medium naval orange, peeled with pith removed

1 cup (235 ml) unsweetened almond milk

5 to 6 ice cubes

Preparation:

In a blender, combine all the ingredients.

Blend on high for 20 seconds or until smooth. Enjoy immediately and slowly sip.

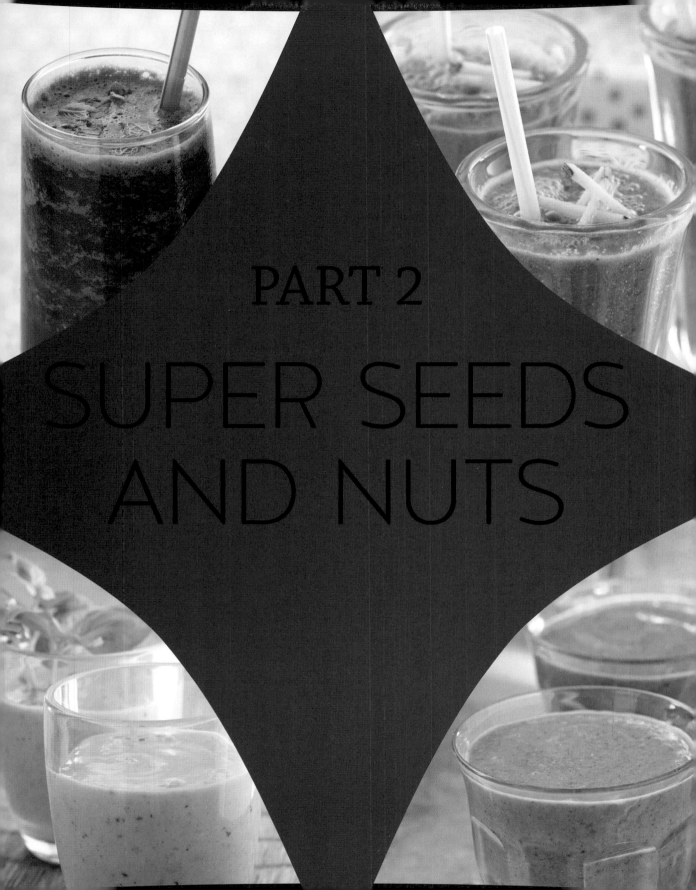

PART 2

SUPER SEEDS AND NUTS

CHAPTER 7

CHIA

AZTEC WARRIOR SUPERFOOD

FEATURED RECIPES

Minty Strawberries and Cream Smoothie

Yin Yang Smoothie

Black Tie Smoothie

Melon Chia Fresca

Spicy Pink Princess Smoothie

Cha-cha-cha-Chia! Yes, it's true, chia seeds are akin to the once, or possibly still, widely popular Chia Pet. Yet these tiny seeds are so much more beneficial to our overall health and well-being when we *consume* them, rather than use them to grow a whimsical pet. You will surely be impressed with how versatile, nutritious, and nutrient-packed this tiny seed is. Because chia is a seed, it is naturally free of allergens associated with nuts, making it a safe snack food for those with food sensitivities.

The edible seeds, derived from the Lamiaceae family of plants grown in Mexico, come with a nutty flavor and a world of nutrition. The word "chia" means "strength" in South American cultures, and

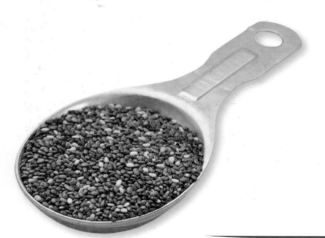

I believe the seeds are named appropriately. These tiny black or white seeds date back to the ancient times when Mayan and Aztec cultures thrived. Warriors of the day consumed chia seeds regularly and abundantly before battle to ensure sustained energy and hydration.

One of the unique properties of the chia seed is its liquid-absorbing capability. When exposed to juice, water, or gastric juices, the tiny seed swells and becomes gelatinous. The consistency promotes a sense of fullness and satiety, slowing the release of dietary sugars into the bloodstream. Chia's gelatinous quality also helps it absorb dietary toxins, fats, and cholesterol, aiding in their elimination.

DYNAMITE DETOXING AGENT

When chia seeds are placed in liquid, including the digestive juices of your stomach, they act like a sponge, soaking it up. This action turns the seeds into an almost sticky and gluelike binding agent that adheres to and helps you effectively eliminate health inhibitors. When you consume chia seeds daily, they act like a resident housekeeper who cleans so frequently your habitat never becomes messy.

In other words, chia is a detox maven! The seeds help to keep the daily toxic load placed on your body in check. Consumption of chia supports the health of your liver, your main detox organ, by gently filtering and metabolizing poisons such as heavy metals, pesticides, food additives, and carcinogens. If your body is flooded with regular doses of liver-supporting nutrients, your elimination systems can function more optimally, resulting in vibrant health. Alternatively, if you do not supplement with vital nutrients such as those you get from chia seeds, your body may become overloaded with many toxins, and your liver may not be able to keep up. What happens then? You hold onto more toxins than you can eliminate and your body becomes a toxic playground. This can lead to a decline in health resulting in digestive troubles, weight gain, bloating, poor skin quality, mental fatigue, and irritability.

HEART-HEALTH FACILITATOR

Chia seeds can help normalize blood sugar levels, reduce inflammation, act as a powerful cell-protecting antioxidant, and contribute to weight loss, which is essential for a healthy heart. Heart disease is the leading cause of death for both men and women in the United States, according to the Centers for Disease Control and Prevention.

One key nutrient in chia that supports heart health is omega-3 fatty acids. Chia seeds, in addition to flaxseeds and walnuts, are a fantastic plant-based source of this polyunsaturated super nutrient, also known as alpha-linolenic acid (ALA). Chia seeds are actually one of the richest plant-based sources of ALA; 1 ounce (28 g) of chia seed contains 9 grams of fat with 75 percent of the total fat coming from ALA!

PROTEIN PACKED AND STAMINA SUSTAINING

You may not think of chia seeds when looking for a protein-dense meal, but you should. One reason chia seeds are so helpful in creating a sense of fullness and improving and sustaining energy is their

mighty nutritional makeup. Just 2 tablespoons (26 g) of chia seeds contain 139 calories, 4 grams of protein, 9 grams of fat, 12 grams of carbohydrates, and 11 grams of fiber, plus vitamins and minerals such as calcium, phosphorus, magnesium, manganese, copper, iron, niacin, and zinc. According to Roxanne B. Sukol, MD, MS, and Brenda Powell, MD, of Cleveland Clinic Wellness, to achieve maximum benefit, follow the dosage recommended by the manufacturer, which on average is 2 tablespoons (26 g), when preparing a chia dish or beverage.

Sourcing and Care of Chia

To create nutritious chia gel, which is perfect for adding to hundreds of recipes, soak the seeds first! Specifically, soak 2 tablespoons (26 g) of chia seeds in 3 to 4 ounces (90 to 120 ml) of liquid for 5 minutes. There is no need to grind chia, and as with most seeds, you can sprout them if desired. When purchasing the seeds, make sure they do not smell rancid. Store in the refrigerator after the packaging they're in has been opened or in a cool, dark, and dry environment such as your pantry. When stored properly, chia will remain fresh for up to one year.

The chef in you will appreciate chia's culinary versatility. It is an excellent thickening and emulsifying agent, adding rich texture and silkiness when blended into smoothies, desserts, and dressings.

✦MINTY STRAWBERRIES✦ AND CREAM SMOOTHIE

You may not know this, but mint and strawberries are super compatible. The mint enhances the sweetness of the berries and adds vibrancy and depth when blended into this nourishing shake. Mint provides more than just good taste; it aids in digestion and contains vitamin D3, which is essential for calcium absorption. Strawberries are rich in iron, which strengthens the blood and enhances absorption of nutrients into your cells. Chia seeds deliver a welcome balance of fat, fiber, and protein and also add silkiness and density to this smoothie as do creamy avocado and coconut milk.

Time: 5 minutes

Equipment: Blender

Yield: Approximately one 20-ounce (570 ml) smoothie

Ingredients:
5 frozen strawberries
¼ medium avocado, peeled and pitted
3 pitted medjool dates
1 small handful fresh mint
½ teaspoon vanilla extract
1 tablespoon (8 g) chia seeds
1½ cups (355 ml) coconut milk
5 to 6 ice cubes

Preparation:
In a blender, combine all the ingredients.

Blend on high for 20 seconds or until smooth. Enjoy immediately and sip slowly.

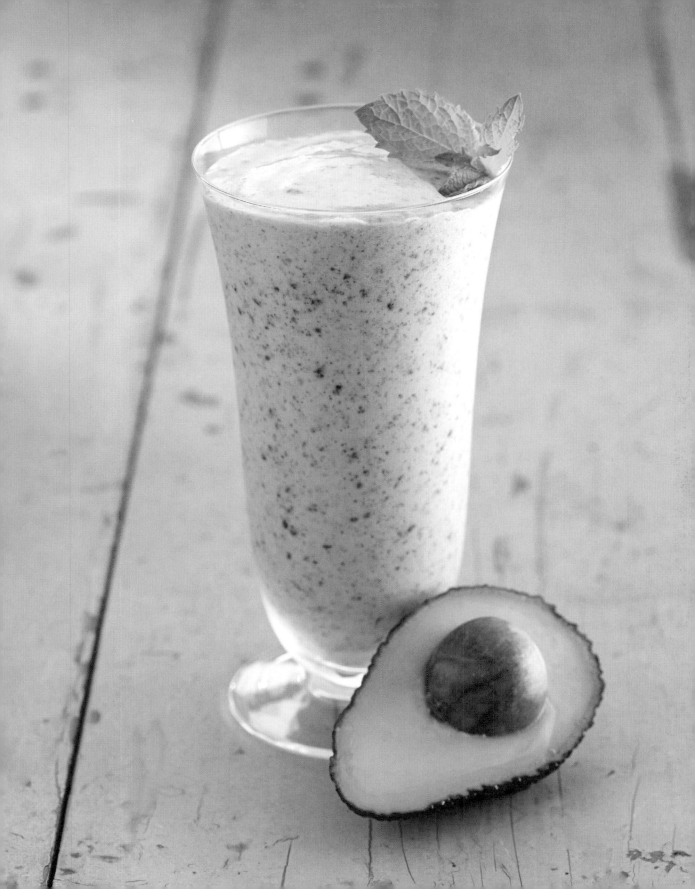

✦YIN YANG SMOOTHIE✦

The natural sugars in the mixed berries fuse with the high fiber, protein, and fat content of chia seeds. This union of nutrients promises a healthy match made in heaven, a yin yang of breakfast delights. The berries are full of antioxidants that beautify your body, promote heart health, and ward off infections and disease. They are also rich in dietary fiber, which keeps your intestines and colon healthy and functioning optimally. Coconut water is loaded with potassium, an essential mineral for maintaining hydration of your tissues and organs, and the addition of greens delivers vitamins and minerals that make your skin glow, whiten your teeth, and detoxify your cells.

Time: 5 minutes

Equipment: Blender

Yield: Approximately one 20-ounce (570 ml) smoothie

Ingredients:
3 kale leaves, de-ribbed and chopped
1 large handful spinach
½ cup (75 g) frozen mixed berries
2 cups (475 ml) coconut water
1 tablespoon (8 g) chia seeds

Preparation:
In a blender, combine all the ingredients.

Blend on high for 20 seconds or until smooth. Enjoy immediately and sip slowly.

✦BLACK TIE SMOOTHIE✦

This is the black tie affair of blended smoothies, deeply detoxifying and delicious. Antioxidant-rich blueberries support resistance to toxic free radicals and mingle gregariously with omega-3-rich chia seeds, intoxicating cacao, aromatic vanilla, and immune-boosting coconut milk. Dates add natural sweetness and fiber, kale offers bone-building vitamin K and calcium, and avocado gives you an abundance of potassium. The result of these ingredients carrying on together is a velvety, chocolaty, berry party.

Time: 5 minutes

Equipment: Blender

Yield: Approximately one 20-ounce (570 ml) smoothie

Ingredients:
½ cup (75 g) fresh or frozen blueberries

4 kale leaves, de-ribbed and chopped

¼ medium avocado, peeled and pitted

1 tablespoon (8 g) chia seeds

3 pitted medjool dates

1 tablespoon (6 g) raw cacao powder

1 teaspoon vanilla extract

1½ cups (355 ml) coconut milk

1 teaspoon cacao nibs

Preparation:
In a blender, combine the blueberries, kale, avocado, chia seeds, dates, cacao powder, vanilla, and coconut milk.

Blend on high for 20 seconds or until smooth.

Pour into a serving glass, sprinkle with cacao nibs, and enjoy.

✦MELON CHIA FRESCA✦

A fresca is a popular drink among people of Mexican and South American cultures. The beverage usually consists of either a blend of fresh fruit juices and diced fruit or juice combined with chia seeds. The tasty concoctions do not only impart a juicy and sweet succulent flavor, they also promote well-being with their nourishing and vitalizing nutrients. In this melon variation, I've selected watermelon for its intoxicating sugary flavor, which plays oh so well with fresh mint and tangy lime.

Time: 25 minutes

Equipment: Blender, small glass jar, and large glass jar

Yield: Approximately two 12-ounce (355 ml) frescas

Ingredients:

¼ cup (60 ml) water

2 teaspoons (5 g) chia seeds

1½ cups (225 g) seedless watermelon, rough chopped

1 cup (235 ml) coconut water

½ lime, juiced

1 small handful fresh mint

8 ice cubes

Preparation:

In a small glass jar, combine the water and chia seeds and let rest for ten minutes. Stir and allow to rest ten minutes more.

Meanwhile, in a blender, combine the watermelon, coconut water, lime juice, mint, and ice.

Blend on high for 20 seconds. Transfer to a large jar. Stir in the chia seeds with their soaking water. Divide between two glasses. Enjoy immediately and sip slowly.

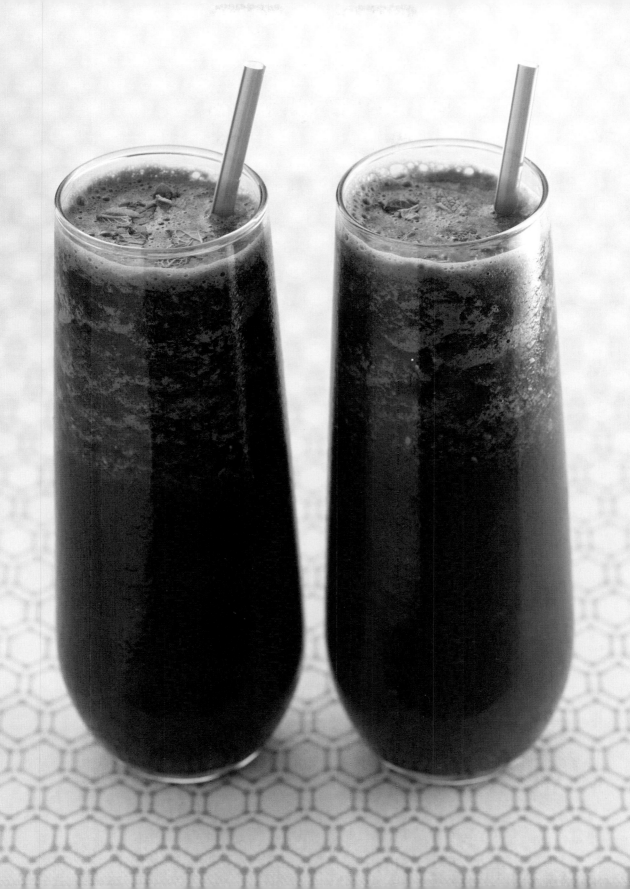

✦SPICY PINK PRINCESS✦ SMOOTHIE

Savory and sweet, this refreshing summertime smoothie is blushing from its charming flavor and nutrient profile. Its balance of carbohydrates from naturally sweet watermelon and fat- and protein-dense chia keeps you feeling energized and sated for hours. Ginger reduces inflammation and bloating in the body, while cilantro supports bone health and adds savor to the flavorful blend. Jalapeño imparts zip and zest as well as heart health support, and the hint of lime has antibacterial properties, warding off disease and infections.

Time: 5 minutes

Equipment: Blender

Yield: Approximately one 20-ounce (570 ml) smoothie

Ingredients:

1 cup (150 g) seedless water-melon, rough chopped

2 sprigs cilantro

1 piece (½ inch, or 1 cm) fresh ginger, peeled

1 tablespoon (8 g) chia seeds

½ lime, juiced

½ small jalapeño, seeds removed

4 pitted medjool dates

1 cup (235 ml) coconut water

Pinch sea salt

Preparation:

In a blender, combine all the ingredients.

Blend on high for 20 seconds or until smooth. Enjoy immediately and sip slowly.

CHAPTER 8

HEMP
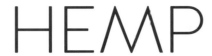

THE HEART-HEALTHY SUPERFOOD

FEATURED RECIPES

Creamy Carrot Stick Smoothie

Blue Genes Smoothie

The Hempty Dance Smoothie

Spiced Choco Pod Smoothie

Vanilla Velvet Smoothie

Although hemp seeds come from the same plant species as marijuana (*Cannabis sativa*), they are extracted from a special variety that does not contain tetrahydrocannabinol (THC), the phyto compound that induces marijuana's psychoactive effects.

A TRULY PERFECT PROTEIN

Instead, these nutritous seeds are a complete protein, one that contains all nine essential amino acids and delivers them in the sufficient quantity and ratio our bodies require. What is especially beneficial about this itty-bitty seed, and others like it such as chia and flax, is that these essential amino acids are present in a single chain format, meaning they don't have to be broken down by enzymes first in order to be digested.

Meat proteins, on the other hand, are full of tangled, long-chain amino acids that must first be broken down into single chains before they can be assimilated and absorbed. This greatly slows and burdens the digestive system, causing indigestion, gas, sensations of heaviness in the gut, sluggishness, and even sleepiness after eating. Hemp protein is so bioavailable (highly digestible) that it gets absorbed and converted into energy right away, stimulating the body and quickly working to provide a number of amazing functions.

A TRULY HEART-HEALTHY FAT

The fatty acid ratio of this super seed is, according to the World Health Organization (WHO), perfect. WHO and health experts such as Mark Hyman, MD, and Joseph Mercola, DO, say the ideal ratio of omega-3 to omega-6 fatty acids is 3:1. The ratio in the Standard American Diet (SAD) is closer to 20:1! According to the University of Maryland Medical Center, that lopsided ratio puts eaters at risk of developing inflammatory diseases such as diabetes, heart disease, and Alzheimer's.

Why do we want omega-3s? The molecular structure of this essential fatty acid has blood-thinning

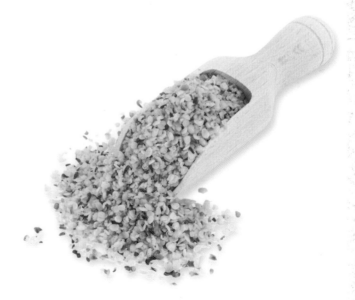

properties, which allows the fats to circulate through the body efficiently. As they do, they reduce the risk of stroke by keeping the paths of arteries clear, preventing hardening, and slowing plaque development.

You want to stay as close to a 3:1 ratio as possible while ensuring the omega-6 you consume is of high quality like that found in hemp. It contains the fat called gamma-linolenic acid (GLA). When consumed, GLA is converted to a substance called dihomo-y-linolenic acid (DGLA), which fights inflammation. An article updated June 4, 2013, from the University of Maryland Medical Center said that consuming GLA fats for six months or more may reduce symptoms of inflammatory disease, such as nerve pain in patients with diabetic neuropathy.

In addition, five researchers at the Wake Forest Center for Botanical Lipids and Inflammatory Disease Prevention in Winston-Salem, North Carolina, studied the effects that dietary supplementation of GLA has on inflammation-induced cardiovascular disease. In their report, they affirm a healthy balance of omega-3 fatty acids with GLA omega-6 affects the biochemistry of fatty acid metabolism and reduces the risk of deadly heart disease.

A HANDFUL OF HEMP VARIETIES

Hemp seeds, hemp protein powder, cold-pressed hemp oil, hemp butter, which is made from ground hemp seeds, and hemp milk made from blended hemp seeds and water are all products that will deeply nourish you, provide energy, and promote vibrant health.

I often use hemp protein powder in my smoothies and to stir into hot buckwheat or quinoa cereal. It has the most deliciously sweet and nutty taste, and one serving (about ¼ cup, or 30 g) provides about 15 g of easily digestible protein and 7 grams of fiber!

In addition to enhancing smoothies and cereals, hemp adds a nutty flavor and hearty texture to baked goods. Use ¾ cup (95 g) flour and ¼ cup (30 g) hemp protein powder for every 1 cup (125 g) of flour called for in a recipe. Your baked goods and treats will turn out a bit denser, but that's a good thing! You'll enjoy nutrient-rich ingredients that will quell cravings and stave off hunger for hours!

Hemp seeds, also known as hemp hearts, are excellent for thickening and emulsifying dressings and sauces. The seeds come at a pretty hefty price (between $17 and $19 per pound on average) so look for them in bulk bins to save on cost. Also keep in mind that in terms of nutritive benefit, just a little bit goes a long way. Just 1 to 2 tablespoons (8 to 15 g) per day is plenty for enhancing your health!

Sourcing and Care of Hemp

When purchasing hemp protein powder, look for varieties that are non-GMO, 100 percent organic, raw, and cold-milled. Refrigerate after opening and use within six months of your first use.

The hemp oil you buy should always be raw, organic, and cold-pressed and purchased from the refrigerated section of your market. Transport it to your refrigerator as soon as possible, and once opened, I suggest you use it within three months to ensure optimum freshness.

Hemp seeds, even in bulk, should also be found in the refrigerator section of your natural food store. If not, do not buy them. They should be kept cool at all times. Store in airtight glass (preferably dark glass) and use within eight to twelve weeks of the purchase date.

✦CREAMY CARROT STICK✦ SMOOTHIE

This smoothie is nutrient dense yet still has a magnificently sweet flavor that both adults and kids will enjoy. The carrot juice, in addition to offering energy-boosting natural sugars, is full of beautifying vitamin A. This essential vitamin brings a healthy glow to your skin, strengthens hair and nails, and brightens your eyes. Spinach, among dozens of other health benefits, offers vitamin K, a necessary nutrient for the growth and strength of your bones. Dates boost the smoothie's sweetness and have adequate amounts of the B complex group of nutrients to regulate mood and your nervous system. Hemp seeds and hemp milk ensure you are nourished and satisfied for hours because of their high protein, fat, and fiber content.

Time: 5 minutes

Equipment: Blender

Yield: Approximately one 20-ounce (570 ml) smoothie

Ingredients:
1½ cups (355 ml) fresh-pressed carrot juice

1 tablespoon (8 g) hemp seeds

1 cup (235 ml) unsweetened hemp milk

2 large handfuls spinach

3 pitted medjool dates

5 to 6 ice cubes

Preparation:
In a blender, combine all the ingredients.

Blend on high for 20 seconds. Enjoy immediately and sip slowly.

✦BLUE GENES SMOOTHIE✦

Get ready for a hearty breakfast smoothie that will stave off hunger until lunchtime. Super antioxidant-rich blueberries are also incredibly high in fiber, helping you to feel pleasantly full for hours. Hemp protein delivers almost 15 grams of complete small chain amino acids and 5 grams of fiber. Medjool dates sweeten lightly and offer up body-calming and tissue-repairing magnesium and blood-supporting iron. Hemp seeds provide heart-healthy omega-3 and omega-6 fats in addition to protein, fiber, and a complementary nutty taste. Drink up daily and your genes will thank you!

Time: 10 minutes

Equipment: Blender

Yield: Approximately one 20-ounce (570 ml) smoothie

Ingredients:

½ cup (75 g) fresh or frozen blueberries

1½ cups (355 ml) unsweetened almond milk

½ cup (120 ml) water

3 tablespoons (23 g) plain or vanilla hemp protein powder

3 pitted medjool dates

½ teaspoon hemp seeds

Preparation:

In a blender, combine the blueberries, almond milk, water, hemp protein powder, and dates.

Blend on high for 20 seconds.

Transfer to a serving glass, sprinkle with hemp seeds, and enjoy!

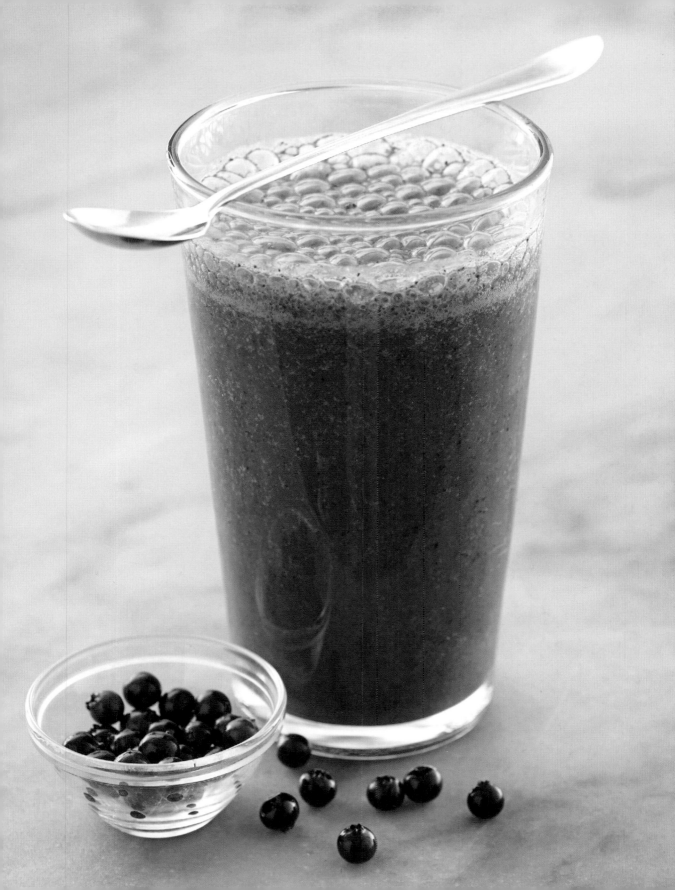

✦THE HEMPTY DANCE✦ SMOOTHIE

Another kid-friendly smoothie, this one is sweetened with whole apple and fresh apple juice. Apple polyphenols help prevent spikes in blood sugar and quercetin, a flavonoid abundant in apples, is excellent for warding off seasonal allergies. Avocado adds a creamy texture to this nutrient powerhouse and offers more potassium, ounce for ounce, than banana. Kale is rich in calcium and contains more of this essential mineral per calorie than dairy milk! And parsley contains a unique anti-oxidant, luteolin, that finds and destroys free radicals in the body. The flavor is so sweet and refreshing, you just might bust out in a little dance!

Time: 5 minutes

Equipment: Blender

Yield: Approximately one 20-ounce (570 ml) smoothie

Ingredients:
½ medium semisweet apple (such as Gala or Fuji)
¼ medium avocado
1 cup (235 ml) fresh-pressed apple juice
½ cup (120 ml) water
2 large kale leaves, de-ribbed
1 large handful spinach
1 small handful parsley
5 to 6 ice cubes
1 teaspoon hemp seeds
Apple slivers, for garnish

Preparation:
In a blender, combine the apple, avocado, apple juice, water, kale, spinach, parsley, and ice.

Blend on high for 20 seconds.

Transfer to a serving glass, stir in the hemp seeds, garnish with apple slivers, and enjoy!

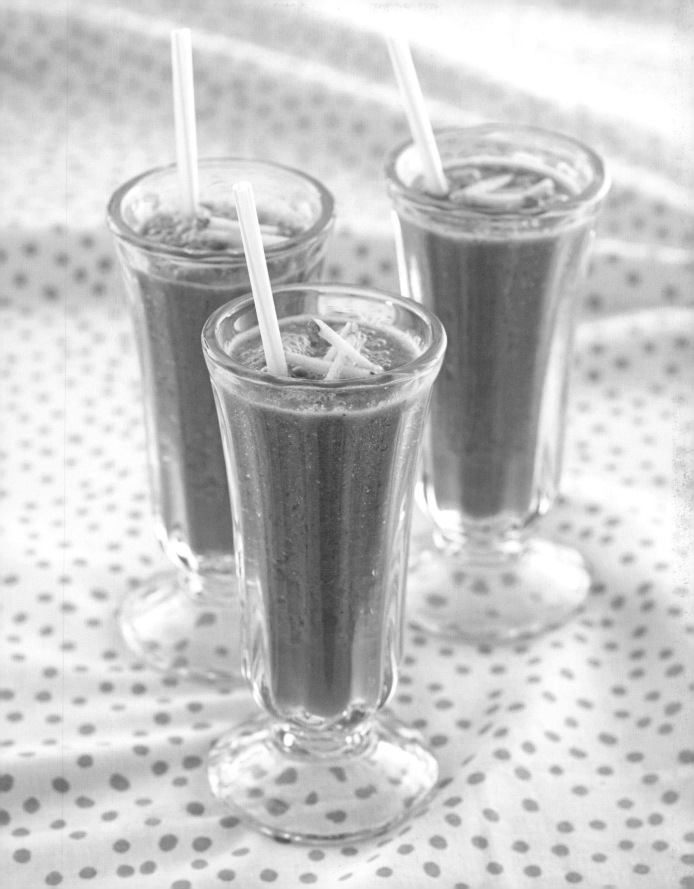

✦SPICED CHOCO POD✦ SMOOTHIE

If you like Mexican hot cacao, you'll love this cooler version! Banana provides a thick and creamy base for this smoothie and an abundance of potassium, an essential mineral for maintaining healthy blood pressure. Chocolate hemp protein powder not only boosts the flavor of this any-time shake, it provides protein necessary for healthy tissue repair. The warming spices of cardamom, cinnamon, nutmeg, and cayenne combine with the chocolate flavor magnificently and stimulate metabolic function. (Can you say: burn calories while you sip?) And last but not least, a touch of hemp oil reduces inflammation in the body and promotes heart health. That deserves a cha-cha-cha if you ask me!

Time: 5 minutes

Equipment: Blender

Yield: Approximately one 20-ounce (570 ml) smoothie

Ingredients:
½ medium banana

1½ cups (355 ml) unsweet-
    ened hemp milk

3 tablespoons (23 g) chocolate
    hemp protein powder

⅛ teaspoon ground cardamom

¼ teaspoon ground cinnamon

⅛ teaspoon ground nutmeg

Small pinch cayenne pepper

1 teaspoon hemp oil

Preparation:
In a blender, combine all the ingredients.

Blend on high for 20 seconds. Enjoy and savor!

✦VANILLA VELVET✦ SMOOTHIE

Sometimes it's fun to have a creamy vanilla treat just like the ice cream we enjoyed as kids. This simple concoction is cool, smooth, sweet, and surprisingly nutritious. Coconut water is a natural electrolyte, making this an ideal shake to enjoy after a workout. The bioavailable protein in the hemp powder is delivered in its most effective form to promote post-workout tissue repair. A touch of sea salt helps to restore salts lost through perspiration, and hemp seeds deliver fat and fiber that will whisk your hunger pains away.

Time: 5 minutes

Equipment: Blender

Yield: Approximately one 20-ounce (570 ml) smoothie

Ingredients:
1 cup (235 ml) coconut milk
1 cup (235 ml) coconut water
3 tablespoons (23 g) vanilla hemp protein powder
1 teaspoon vanilla extract
Pinch sea salt
10 ice cubes
1 teaspoon hemp seeds

Preparation:
In a blender, combine the coconut milk and water, hemp protein, vanilla extract, sea salt, and ice.

Blend on high for 20 seconds.

Transfer to a serving glass, sprinkle with hemp seeds, and enjoy!

CHAPTER 9

FLAX

BRAIN-BOOSTING SUPER SEED

FEATURED RECIPES

Matcha Maker Smoothie

Turmeric Mango Lassi

Flax 'n' Berry Smoothie

Zucchini Bread Smoothie

Pure Braun Smoothie

Flax, also known as linseed, has a Latin name of *Linum usitatissimum*. This translates to "most useful," and I couldn't agree more. Flax is not only a culinary catch, it is also useful in nourishing the body and protecting against some very gnarly health foes. Consumption of the tiny brown and golden seeds dates back as far as 3000 BCE when it was cultivated in Babylon. Charlemagne, who reined in the eighth century as King of the Franks, so deeply believed in its health power that he passed laws requiring the people he governed to eat it.

A HEART HEALTH HERO

Modern research shows that eating flaxseeds as a dietary supplement can reduce depression, combat cancer, support heart health, reduce the risk of brain disease, and promote digestive regularity. The nutrients responsible for these health benefits are fiber and omega-3 and omega-6 fatty acids. Like hemp seeds, flax contains the ideal omega-3 to 6 ratio of 3:1. This proper balance of acids works to form the membranes and support healthy function of all cells in your body.

Tanya Quod, national naturopathy chair for the Australian Natural Therapists Association, says the acids in flaxseed help to lower blood pressure and LDL (bad) cholesterol, thus reducing the risk of cardiovascular disease. In a study conducted at the University

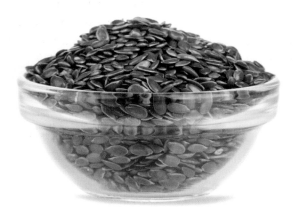

Eat Flax for Regularity

Eating ground flaxseed works wonders in keeping you regular and preventing constipation. The fiber in flaxseed binds with water and swells to form a gel. This gel helps to soften stool and gently moves it through your intestines. This is only achieved with flax powder, not the oil from which all the fiber has been extracted.

of Toronto, a group of nine women ate 50 grams of milled flaxseed each day for four weeks in addition to their regular diet. After four weeks, their total cholesterol levels had decreased 9 percent and their LDL (bad) cholesterol had dropped 18 percent.

In addition, omega-3 fatty acids, also known as alpha-linolenic acid (ALA), thin our blood, helping to prevent blood clots and reduce the risk of stroke. In October 2007, five researchers at Harokopio University's Department of Nutrition and Dietetics in Athens, Greece, studied the effects of flaxseed oil consumption on participants with high blood pressure. They found that daily supplementation of the omega-3-rich oil significantly lowered systolic and diastolic blood pressure levels. Further, the *Nurses' Health Study,* which commenced in 1980, followed 76,000 women through the year 2000. Those who consumed the most ALA cut their risk of dying from a fatal heart attack in half. Whole flaxseeds and oil contain far more ALA than many other foods.

BOLD BRAIN POWER BOOSTER

Since nearly 60 percent of our brain is made of lipids (fats), omega-3-rich foods support the health of brain tissue. In addition, ALAS are known to improve the function of the cerebral cortex, the area that processes sensory information such as taste and touch.

Udo Erasmus, PhD, says flax has a mood-boosting ingredient called docosahexaenoic acid (DHA) that is essential for the healthy function of brain cells. Martha Clare Morris, MD, of Rush-Presbyterian-St. Luke's Medical Center in Chicago suggests that eating omega-3 fatty acids is paramount to brain development and health. In a seven-year study, which commenced in 1993, she saw the risk of developing Alzheimer's disease reduced by 60 percent in subjects between ages 65 and 94 who regularly consumed omega-3 fatty acids.

FLAX FLAVOR AND VERSATILITY

The taste of flax is one of pleasant nuttiness. It harmoniously integrates with sweet, salty, and savory foods, making it a joyful addition to smoothies, desserts, soups, stews, breakfast cereals, and crackers. It can even be used as an egg substitute for binding ingredients in breads, muffins, and veggie burgers. The ratio of water to flax meal is 3:1, and the quantity needed for every egg called for in a recipe is 3 tablespoons (45 ml) of water to 1 tablespoon (14 g) flax meal. Stir to combine and let rest for two minutes. When using flax as an egg substitute, your resulting baked goods and burgers will have a slightly chewier and denser texture.

To introduce flax into your diet, begin with 2 teaspoons (5 g) of ground flax and work up to 2 tablespoons (14 g) per day. To get your daily quota of omega-3s, try 1½ teaspoons of flax oil, which contains a recommended 4 grams.

✦MATCHA MAKER✦ SMOOTHIE

Matcha, a finely milled green tea powder, is used in Japanese tea ceremonies. Drinking matcha delivers far more nutrients to your system than sipping common green tea. When you drink matcha, you are drinking the ground whole leaf as opposed to just the brewed tea achieved by steeping the leaves. Matcha is extremely high in antioxidant content, and, as discovered by Tufts University researchers, is significantly higher in antioxidants than pomegranates or blueberries. It has a naturally robust and nutty flavor, which marries harmoniously with coconut. Though it does contain caffeine, the amount in this smoothie is only one-fourth of that of a 12-ounce (355 ml) cup of coffee. In addition, the caffeine in matcha has an alkalinizing effect on the body rather than an acidic response like that of coffee and colas. The slightly "green" taste of the matcha is delicately balanced with sweet fresh dates, creamy coconut milk, maple syrup, and vanilla. Flax adds a delicate nutty flavor and delivers essential fatty acids to ensure your teatime is packed with brain-nourishing nutrients.

Time: 5 minutes

Equipment: Blender

Yield: Approximately one 16-ounce (475 ml) smoothie

Ingredients:
1 tablespoon (5 g) coconut flakes
2 teaspoons (5 g) flax meal
1 teaspoon matcha tea powder
½ teaspoon vanilla extract
2 pitted medjool dates
1 teaspoon maple syrup
1 cup (235 ml) coconut milk
1 cup (235 ml) water

Preparation:
In a blender, combine all the ingredients.

Blend on high for 20 seconds or until smooth. Enjoy immediately and sip slowly.

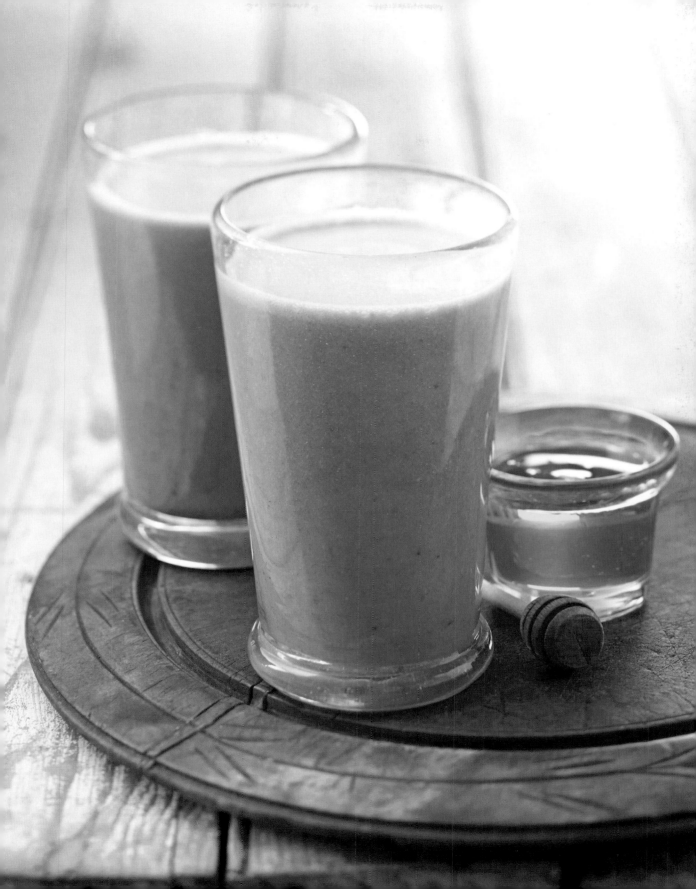

+TURMERIC MANGO LASSI+

Turmeric and fresh ginger are incredible digestive aids and have potent anti-inflammatory properties. Adding them to your diet can support bowel regularity, soothe indigestion, and reduce arthritic pain and muscle aches. They are also powerful immune boosters. Sweet mango contains tartaric and malic acids, which promote body alkalinity. We want a more alkaline pH in the body to ward off infections and disease. Creamy and decadent coconut yogurt and milk marry perfectly with tropical mango, sugary banana, and dates. Ground flax meal adds silkiness and density, resulting in a refreshing and luscious Indian-inspired health shake.

Time: 5 minutes

Equipment: Blender

Yield: Approximately one 20-ounce (570 ml) lassi

Ingredients:

1 container (6 ounce or 170 g) coconut yogurt (plain or vanilla)

½ medium banana

2 pitted medjool dates

½ cup (90 g) frozen mango chunks

1 piece (½ inch, or 1 cm) fresh ginger, peeled

½ teaspoon ground turmeric

2 teaspoons (5 g) ground flax meal

1 cup (235 ml) coconut milk

Preparation:

In a blender, combine all the ingredients.

Blend on high for 20 seconds or until smooth. Enjoy immediately and sip slowly.

✦FLAX 'N' BERRY SMOOTHIE✦

Simple and bursting with heart-protecting, brain-boosting, and digestion-supporting goodness, this smoothie is both delicious and nutritious! Strawberries have huge antioxidant power and an abundance of immunity-aiding and muscle-loving vitamin C. Flax oil delivers omega-3 fatty acids, and a kiss of maple syrup adds subtle sweetness.

Time: 5 minutes

Equipment: Blender

Yield: Approximately one 20-ounce (570 ml) smoothie

Ingredients:
½ medium banana

1 cup (225 g) frozen strawberries

1 tablespoon (7 g) ground flax

1 teaspoon flax oil

1½ cups (355 ml) unsweetened vanilla almond milk

1 teaspoon maple syrup

Preparation:
In a blender, combine all the ingredients.

Blend on high for 20 seconds or until smooth. Enjoy immediately and sip slowly.

+ZUCCHINI BREAD+ SMOOTHIE

This delectable smoothie tastes just like zucchini bread but can be enjoyed without guilt. Full of fiber, protein, and healthy fat, it will sustain you for hours, making it an excellent breakfast option. Zucchini is rich in magnesium, and one serving contains 40 percent of the RDA of manganese, which supports the metabolization of proteins and carbohydrates. Gluten-free oats provide fiber and density, and the warming spices of cinnamon, nutmeg, and clove act as anti-inflammatories. The addition of almond butter not only boosts the delicious zucchini bread flavor, its monounsaturated fats also support heart health and reduce LDL (bad) cholesterol levels.

Time: 5 minutes

Equipment: Blender

Yield: Approximately one 20-ounce (570 ml) smoothie

Ingredients:

1 small zucchini, ends trimmed, chopped

½ medium banana

2 pitted medjool dates

¼ teaspoon ground cinnamon

⅛ teaspoon ground nutmeg

¼ cup (20 g) gluten-free oats

1 tablespoon (15 g) almond butter

2 teaspoons (5 g) ground flax

Pinch of ground cloves

Pinch of sea salt

1 cup (235 ml) unsweetened almond milk

½ cup (120 ml) water

Preparation:

In a blender, combine all the ingredients.

Blend on high for 20 seconds or until smooth. Enjoy immediately and sip slowly.

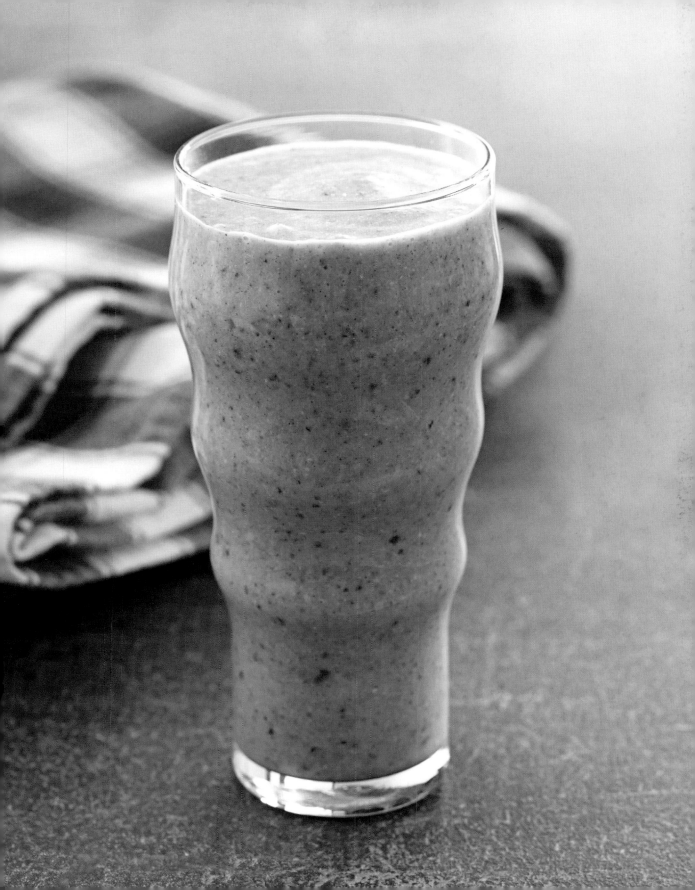

✦PURE BRAUN SMOOTHIE✦

Get your greens and omega-3s in this tasty and nutrient-dense smoothie. Spinach and romaine lettuce provide antioxidants, an abundance of bone-strengthening calcium, and plenty of vitamin C, which is excellent for immunity and tissue repair. Plant-based protein helps to build muscle mass and keeps you feeling fuller longer as does the fiber-rich flax meal. Flax oil provides you with your daily required intake of heart- and brain-nourishing omega-3 fatty acids. The bite of the greens gently slips into the background, masked by sweet banana, coconut water, and vanilla-flavored protein powder, leaving a pleasant taste dancing on your palette.

Time: 5 minutes

Equipment: Blender

Yield: Approximately one 20-ounce (570 ml) smoothie

Ingredients:

½ medium banana

2 tablespoons (15 g) vanilla plant protein powder (such as pea or hemp)

1 handful spinach

3 large romaine leaves

½ cup (120 ml) coconut milk

1½ cups (355 ml) coconut water

2 teaspoons (5 g) flax meal

1 teaspoon flax oil

Preparation:

In a blender, combine all the ingredients.

Blend on high for 20 seconds or until smooth. Enjoy immediately and sip slowly.

CHAPTER 10

SACHA INCHI

OMEGA-3 POWER SEED

FEATURED RECIPES
The Warrior Smoothie
Mighty Mint Smoothie
Matcha Sacha Milk Shake
Malted Maca Inchi Shake
Union Smoothie

Sacha inchi seeds, also called mountain peanuts and Inca peanuts, are a staple in the Peruvian diet. From a hearty vine, buds beautiful star-shaped pods containing four to seven sacha seeds. The pod fruit is not edible, but the seeds are and have extraordinary health properties. They are one of the many foods associated with the excellent health and longevity of the Andean people.

A CONVENIENT COMPLETE PROTEIN

Sacha inchi seeds are called mountain peanuts in South America because despite being true seeds, their texture, size, and flavor are more like that of a roasted peanut. They are considered a complete protein, meaning they contain all essential amino acids in small-chain (the most easily digestible) form. In 1 ounce (28 g), about a small handful, there are 8 grams of protein, making them a convenient and valuable source of this essential macronutrient.

A healthy and strong body requires protein synthesis for tissue repair, muscle strength and development, organ function, and many other bodily functions. According to T. Colin Campbell, MD,

John McDougall, MD, and other nutrition and health experts, an ideal percentage of protein per day is 10 percent of your total calories. So if you were to consume 2,000 calories in a day, that equates to 200 protein calories.

SACHA INCHI FOR BRAIN AND HEART HEALTH

Sacha inchi are also brimming with essential fatty acids, which contribute to brain and heart health. As you learned earlier, the ideal omega-3 to omega-6 ratio is 3:1. These delicious and crunchy seeds contain both in the proper ratio and have gained popularity because of this quality. Having a proper balance of the two acids is what keeps blood circulating throughout the body, protects against clogging of the arteries, and contributes to optimum blood flow to the brain, enhancing mental acuity.

It is no wonder sacha inchi seeds are a commonly enjoyed food in their native land. It is not often that you come across a single food source so balanced

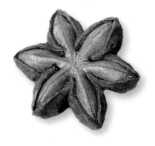
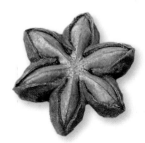

in nutrients. Between their protein and fatty acid content they make a powerfully satisfying addition to anyone's diet. The 27 percent protein content of sacha inchi proves them to be an excellent choice for building strength and muscle tone. Also, more protein means you stay sated longer and have more balanced energy throughout the day.

ANCIENT ANTIDEPRESSANT AIDS IN WEIGHT LOSS

The humble sacha inchi has just recently begun to establish a reputation among nutrition mavens such as Mehmet Oz, MD, for its role in aiding weight loss. The tasty seeds help alleviate hunger because of their ample protein, fat, and fiber, helping us feel fuller longer.

But the most notable reason sacha inchi seeds are being recognized for their contribution to weight loss is their remarkably high level of tryptophan. The seeds contain about 29 mg of this amino acid per gram of protein, which is nearly eight times that of turkey, the most talked about food source of the amino acid. Tryptophan plays a significant role in the production of serotonin, a chemical responsible for regulating mood and contributing to feelings of well-being that's found in the gut and central nervous system. When our mood is regulated, we tend to be happier and less likely to have cravings or overeat. Snacking on sacha inchi can keep your mood in check as well as your appetite.

SACHA INCHI'S BOLD FLAVOR AND USES

Sacha inchi seeds have a taste all their own. I have heard many descriptions but find they are most aptly described as being similar to a combination of flaxseed, peanuts, and Marcona almonds, the latter of which also resemble the sacha inchi in appearance

Sourcing and Care of Sacha Inchi

Sacha Inchi seeds can be found at numerous health food markets and larger retail chains that carry them in sealed bags. They're also readily available through online shops. There are so many sources, in fact, that you may benefit from doing comparison shopping to find the best price. Many companies that sell whole seeds also carry the sacha inchi protein powder.

The care of sacha inchi seeds will differ depending on whether you buy roasted or raw seeds and protein powder. Both plain and flavored toasted seeds are fine to snack on, but the quality of the omega fatty acids declines with cooking. Keep sacha inchi in the cabinet in an airtight bag and reserve the seeds for salad toppings or the occasional snack. Raw sacha inchi seeds should be refrigerated in a sealed container to prevent rancidity and used within four months of purchase. Likewise, sacha inchi protein powder should be refrigerated if you do not anticipate using all of your stock within one month; otherwise, it may be stored in its sealed bag in a cool, dry environment, such as your pantry.

and crunch. Their flavor yields well to nut milks, raw and vegan treats made with dried fruit, dehydrated crackers, and seed pâtes. They also liven green and grain salads, and their protein powder beautifully blends into the background of a variety of smoothies.

✦THE WARRIOR SMOOTHIE✦

Smooth, luscious, and chocolaty may be what you associate with dessert, but I'm talking about a superpowered breakfast with this recipe! You'll be powered by protein with this warrior's morning delight. Cacao provides more than sixty antioxidants and imparts a richness that will bring the whole family to the table for the most important meal of the day. Turn your whole family into weekday warriors with this supremely sumptuous smoothie!

Time: 10 minutes

Equipment: Blender

Yield: Approximately one 20-ounce (570 ml) smoothie

Ingredients:

3 tablespoons (24 g) sacha inchi protein powder

1 medium banana

1½ cups (355 ml) unsweetened almond milk

2 tablespoons (12 g) raw cacao powder

1 teaspoon vanilla extract

⅛ teaspoon sea salt

Preparation:

In a blender, combine all the ingredients.

Blend on high for 20 seconds or until smooth. Serve with a dusting of cacao powder. Enjoy!

✦MIGHTY MINT SMOOTHIE✦

This smoothie includes some of my absolute favorite nutritious foods on the planet. Protein-packed sacha inchi powder ensures that not only do you get sustained energy and muscle support, but that you get a healthy dose of brain-building omega fatty acids to boot! And, as if it couldn't get better than that, I've thrown in one of my all-time adored digestive tonic herbs, our humble and familiar friend, peppermint. Not only is peppermint excellent for stimulating digestion and soothing upset stomachs, it increases circulation, ensuring those smoothie nutrients travel through your bloodstream with efficiency. This is one smoothie to turn to when you need all of your daily nutrition in one straight shot!

Time: 5 minutes

Equipment: Blender

Yield: Approximately one 20-ounce (570 ml) smoothie

Ingredients:

2 tablespoons (16 g) sacha inchi protein powder

2 cups (475 ml) unsweetened hemp or almond milk

1 cup (30 g) fresh spinach leaves

1 medium kale leaf

6 pitted medjool dates

½ medium avocado

10 fresh mint leaves

2 drops peppermint essential oil or ½ teaspoon peppermint extract

Pinch of sea salt

Preparation:

In a blender, combine all the ingredients.

Blend on high for 20 seconds or until smooth. Serve in a tall glass with a sprig of mint.

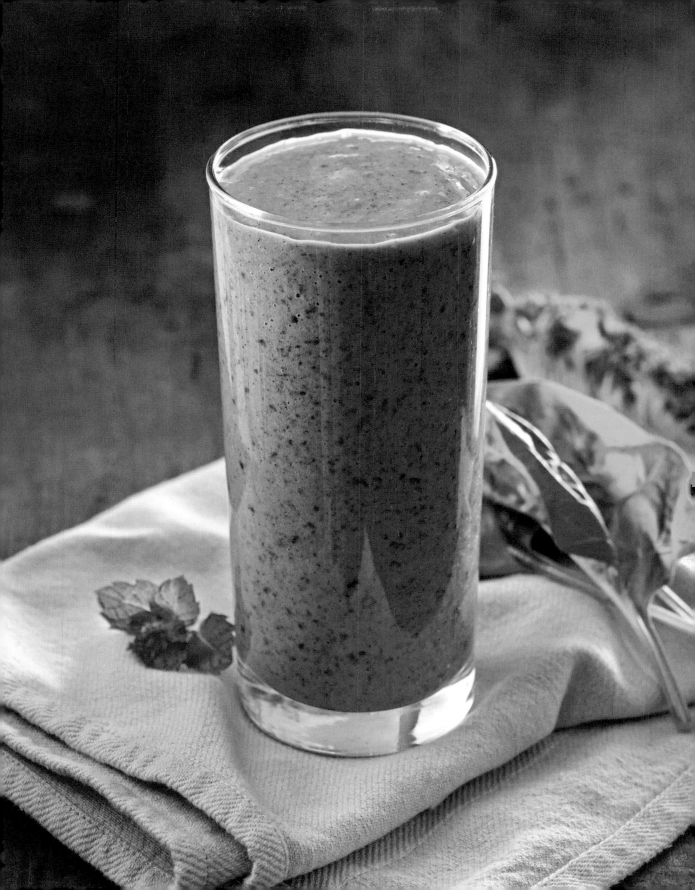

✦MATCHA SACHA✦ MILK SHAKE

You are cordially invited to drink this blend daily to enhance your longevity and give aging the old one-two! Sacha inchi seeds are chock-full of macronutrients, which keep you satisfied for hours, but the antioxidant power of matcha keeps you feeling and looking radiant for the long haul. Its free radical–repelling ability supports youthfulness, a reduction in disease, and contributes to the glow of vibrant health! And even though it does contain caffeine, an amino acid in the tea known as L-theanine has a calming effect and counteracts any jitteriness.

Time: 15 minutes

Equipment: Blender, bowl or pitcher, nut milk bag or fine-mesh strainer, and cheesecloth

Yield: Approximately one 20-ounce (570 ml) milk shake

Ingredients:
½ cup (84 g) sacha inchi seeds
2 cups (475 ml) water
1 tablespoon (8 g) sacha inchi protein powder
¼ medium avocado
2 teaspoons (4 g) matcha powder
5 pitted medjool dates
1 tablespoon (9 g) sunflower seeds

Preparation:
In a blender, combine the sacha inchi seeds and water. Blend until smooth, about one minute.

Line a large bowl or pitcher with a nut milk bag or set in a strainer lined with cheesecloth. Pour through the blended sacha inchi seeds.

Press the sacha inchi milk through the strainer and return to the blender.

Add the protein powder, avocado, matcha powder, dates, and sunflower seeds.

Blend on high for 20 seconds or until completely smooth. Serve cold and enjoy!

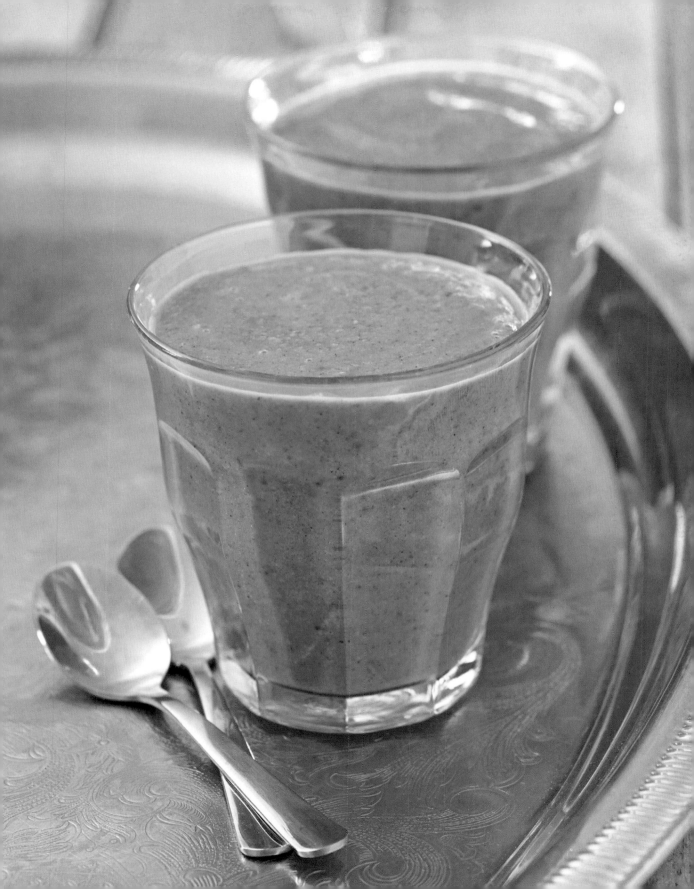

✦MALTED MACA INCHI✦ SHAKE

Many people have a hard time getting going in the morning without a dose of caffeine to bump them out of a sleepy stupor. Others can't touch the stuff without a major case of the jitters. Whether you're trying to cut back on coffee or looking for an alternative early morning power-up, I highly recommend this smooth and creamy confection. Aside from the powerful nutritional kick of sacha inchi seeds, this smoothie also includes a serving of maca, which increases energy levels while supporting your entire endocrine system! That means instead of burning out your adrenals, you could actually support them without missing the extra energy from caffeinated drinks.

Time: 15 minutes

Equipment: Blender, bowl or pitcher, nut milk bag or fine-mesh strainer, and cheesecloth

Yield: Approximately one 20-ounce (570 ml) smoothie

Ingredients:
½ cup (84 g) sacha inchi seeds

2 cups (475 ml) water

1 medium frozen banana

2 teaspoons (10 g) maca powder

1 tablespoon (15 g) lucuma powder

3 pitted medjool dates

1 tablespoon (7 g) green powder (such as spirulina or chlorella)

1 teaspoon vanilla extract

¼ teaspoon sea salt

10 ice cubes

Preparation:
In a blender, combine the sacha inchi seeds and water. Blend until smooth, about one minute.

Line a large bowl or pitcher with a nut milk bag or set in a strainer lined with cheesecloth. Pour through the blended sacha inchi seeds.

Press the sacha inchi milk through the strainer and return to the blender.

Add the frozen banana, maca powder, lucuma powder, dates, green powder, vanilla extract, sea salt, and ice.

Blend on high for 20 seconds or until completely smooth. Serve cold, and enjoy!

✦UNION SMOOTHIE✦

Smoothies are generally called smoothies for a reason. Rich and creamy or silky smooth are the name of the game, but I just love to shake things up a bit when it comes to the classic smoothie paradigm. For this one, I've suggested tossing in some whole sacha inchi seeds to create an unexpected union of creaminess and crunch. As you delight in this decadent blend, your body will adore the brain-tingling effect omega fatty acids impart. Sweet and tangy cherries boost your antioxidant reserves and harmoniously blend with blood sugar–moderating lucuma. They both slide in to complement the flavor of nutty sacha inchi.

Time: 5 minutes

Equipment: Blender

Yield: Approximately one 20-ounce (570 ml) smoothie

Ingredients:
2 tablespoons (16 g) sacha inchi protein powder
1 cup (155 g) fresh or frozen cherries, pitted
1½ cups (355 ml) hemp milk
1 tablespoon (15 g) lucuma powder
1 teaspoon vanilla extract
2 tablespoons (40 g) maple syrup
10 chocolate covered sacha inchi seeds, whole

Preparation:
In a blender, combine the sacha inchi protein powder, cherries, hemp milk, lucuma powder, vanilla extract, and maple syrup.

Blend on high for 20 seconds or until completely smooth.

Pour into a serving glass and stir in the chocolate covered sacha inchi seeds. Enjoy!

CHAPTER 11

COCONUT

THE SUPER FAT

FEATURED RECIPES

Copacabana Smoothie

Sweet and Spicy Smoothie

The Hottie Smoothie

Dream Bar Smoothie

C20 Orange Fresca

You are about to be let in on a secret. I am having a love affair. Yep, that's right . . . with coconut! This love connection began after I recognized that coconut is one of only a few food sources with multiple applications for internal and external use. Not only can it be eaten, coconut can also be used as an effective skin moisturizer, lip balm, and hair conditioner.

Its long list of edible forms includes coconut palm sugar, oil, butter, milk, water, aminos (a soy-free and low-sodium alternative to soy sauce and tamari), flour, meat, and cream. When I discovered all of these yummy forms of coconut and began incorporating them into my diet and cooking, I fell head over heels. As with many love relationships, distance makes the heart grow fonder. Though I'd like to eat it all day long, coconut is still a saturated fat, so I choose to practice moderation. Portion control plus time between mouthwatering engagements equals deep and undying love.

Its multitude of forms and uses is just one reason you may come to love coconut, too. In my opinion, what makes it most attractive is its abundance of health benefits. Did you know that eating coconut can help you lose weight, lower your LDL (bad) cholesterol, and increase your metabolism? It is also known to reduce the risk of heart disease and high blood pressure.

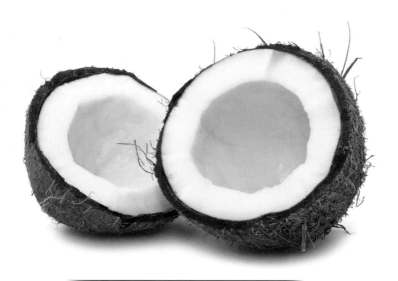

COCONUT COMBATS MULTIPLE HEALTH WOES

Once considered taboo because of its high saturated fat content, we now know that the saturated fat in coconut oil is unique and different from its counterparts. Marisa Moore, a spokeswoman for the American Dietetic Association, has said, "Different types of saturated fats behave differently." The majority of coconut's fat content, 66 percent, is lauric acid, a medium-chain fatty acid (MCFA). All other saturated fats contain long-chain fatty acids (LCFAS), which gum up our blood and get stored as fat. Once ingested, lauric acid converts to monolaurin, a molecule that a number of doctors such as Andrew Weil, MD, and Joseph Mercola, DO, say reduces inflammation in the body and fights infections, bacteria, and viruses.

It's no wonder that Pacific Islanders consider coconut oil to be the cure for all illnesses. The coconut palm is so highly regarded in their culture that they call it the tree of life. Though coconut has been enjoyed and revered around the globe for centuries, only in recent years has modern science discovered its secret healing powers. For example, in April 2002 researchers at Johann-Wolfgang Goethe-Universität in Frankfurt, Germany, discovered coconut oil serves as a suitable wound healer. They say it is effective because of the presence of lauric acid, which acts as an antibacterial and antifungal treatment.

According to researchers at the Universidade Federal de Alagoas in Brazil, coconut oil has the ability to increase our HDL (good) cholesterol and lower our LDL (bad). To arrive at this conclusion, the team conducted a study in 2009 where forty women, ages twenty to forty, were split into two equal groups. The first group received a 30 ml (1 ounce) daily dose of soybean oil and the other twenty women were given a 30 ml (1 ounce) daily dose of coconut oil. Both groups were put on low-calorie, low-carbohydrate diets and were advised to walk fifty minutes every

Sourcing and Care of Coconut

When shopping for coconut oil, choose unrefined virgin varieties. Coconut butter and oil may be stored for two years at room temperature if you can manage to make them last that long. Shredded and flaked coconut as well as coconut flour can often be found in the bulk section of your health food store or packaged in the baking isle. Coconut aminos are usually nestled between soy sauce and tamari on the Asian food aisle of your market.

How much coconut is healthy to consume? Health experts such as Mehmet Oz, MD, and Joseph Mercola, MD, suggest eating up to 3 tablespoons (45 ml) of the virgin oil or butter per day. If you would rather enjoy whole food versions such as unsweetened shredded coconut, coconut milk, or raw meat, aim to keep your intake under ½ cup (40 g) per day.

Cooking with Coconut Oil

Unlike all other concentrated oils, coconut oil is heat stable with a smoke point of about 360°F (182°C). This makes it an ideal oil for cooking and frying. Because of its stability, it is slow to oxidize and thus resistant to rancidity.

Light coconut milk is a welcome addition to puréed soups, such as cream of broccoli, and those made from parsnips, cauliflower, or sweet potatoes. You can achieve creaminess without unnecessary fat and calories. You may, however, want to consider calling on full-fat coconut milk when a touch of decadence is in order.

For a nontraditional twist, you won't regret ditching the dairy to make your own fluffy coconut whip cream. After chilling a 14-ounce (414 ml) can of coconut milk in your refrigerator for at least twelve hours (and ideally overnight), turn the can upside down and remove the bottom with a can opener. The water will have separated from the fat during refrigeration and will be resting on the bottom. Drink the electrolyte-rich water while you make your whip or fill an ice cube mold and use the cubes to not only chill, but sweeten, your next smoothie.

Remaining in the top of the can will be the hardened coconut milk. Quickly spoon it into a mixing bowl and add ½ teaspoon vanilla extract and 1 tablespoon (7 g) yacon syrup. Using a hand mixer, beat the coconut milk into a fluffy whip cream. Use the cream to top desserts, add a dollop to your tea and coffee, or use to enhance the goodness of holiday beverages such as the Anytime Nog (page 44) or the Fall Holiday Smoothie (page 161).

day. At the end of the twelve-week trial, both groups were tested. The group that received the daily dose of coconut oil had elevated levels of HDL and lower overall LDL cholesterol, whereas the group that ingested soybean oil had higher LDL and lower HDL.

EAT FAT TO LOSE WEIGHT

MCFAS, unlike other saturated fats, do not require the engagement of the liver and gallbladder and so are easier to digest. MCFAS, such as those found in coconut, promote a bodily function called *thermogenesis*, which increases our metabolic rate and produces energy much like the conversion of carbohydrates into energy. This increased metabolic rate improves circulation, increases caloric burn, and promotes weight loss.

In July 1989, researchers at the Department of Pediatrics at Vanderbilt University in Nashville, Tennessee, studied the effects of thermogenesis in humans who were overfed medium-chain fatty acids. Ten male volunteers were overfed diets containing 40 percent fat as either MCFA or LCFA. Each participant was studied for one week on each diet. "Our results demonstrate that excess dietary energy as MCFA stimulates thermogenesis to a greater degree than does excess energy as LCFA. This increased energy expenditure provides evidence that excess energy derived from MCFA is stored with a lesser efficiency," the researchers said.

✦COPACABANA SMOOTHIE✦

Think piña colada with a hit of healthy greens. Fresh cucumber adds a cool factor while delivering a heavy dose of zinc, a skin beautifying mineral. Spinach provides you with an abundance of vitamins such as eye-supporting A, immune system–boosting C, and energizing B. Avocado is full of fiber and easily digestible fat. Pineapple contains bromelein, a fruit enzyme that aids in the digestion of protein. It also provides tropical flavor that is known for its harmonious interplay with the sweet and nutty flavor of coconut.

Time: 5 minutes

Equipment: Blender

Yield: Approximately one 20-ounce (570 ml) smoothie

Ingredients:

½ cup (80 g) frozen pineapple bits

¼ cucumber, chopped

1 large handful spinach

2 tablespoons (15 g) vanilla plant protein powder (such as pea or hemp)

¼ medium avocado

1 cup (235 ml) coconut water

1 tablespoon (5 g) unsweetened coconut flakes or shredded coconut

Preparation:

In a blender, combine all the ingredients.

Blend on high for 20 seconds or until smooth. Enjoy immediately and sip slowly.

✦SWEET AND SPICY✦ SMOOTHIE

During travels to Thailand, I loved snacking on fresh mango served with sweet and spicy red chili sauce. Upon my return, I wanted to capture the same flavors but in a nourishing and refreshing shake. This smoothie combines metabolism-revving Thai chili with succulent mango and sweet banana. All are blended with cooling coconut water and creamy coconut milk, which provide natural sugars and heart-healthy fats. Basil adds a savory and complex hint to this unexpectedly delicious smoothie.

Time: 5 minutes

Equipment: Blender

Yield: Approximately one 20-ounce (570 ml) smoothie

Ingredients:

½ cup (90 g) frozen mango chunks

¼ medium avocado

¼ Thai red bird chili or ½ medium red jalapeño, seeds removed (to taste)

3 basil leaves, preferably Thai basil

½ medium banana

½ cup (120 ml) coconut milk

¾ cup (175 ml) coconut water

1 teaspoon shredded unsweetened coconut

Preparation:

In a blender, combine the mango, avocado, chili, Thai basil, banana, coconut milk, and coconut water.

Blend on high for 20 seconds or until smooth.

Transfer to a serving glass and sprinkle with shredded coconut. Enjoy immediately and sip slowly.

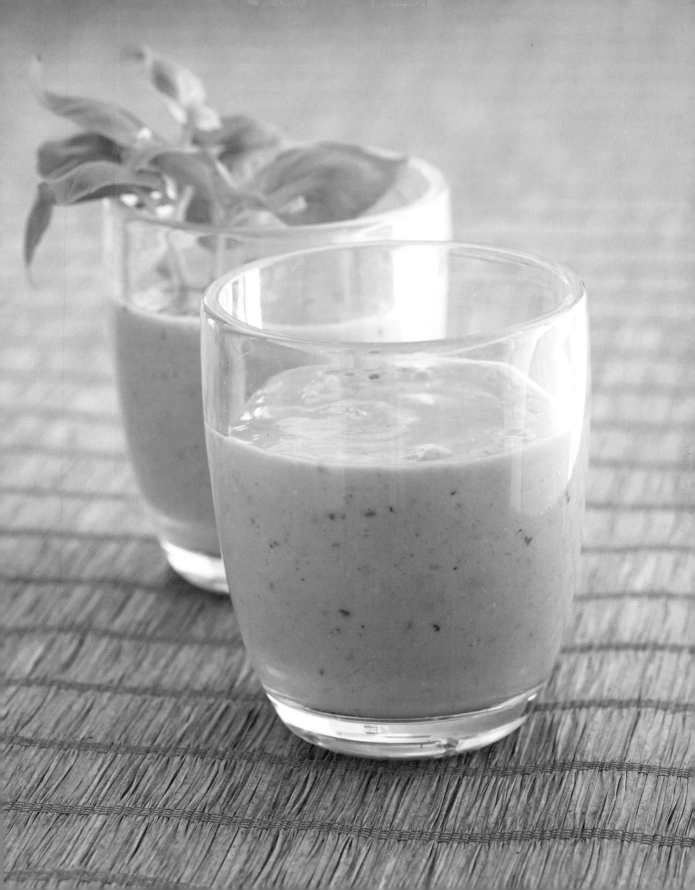

✦THE HOTTIE SMOOTHIE✦

This creamy delight has some serious kick! Not only does jalapeño impart a unique flavor burst to accompanying sweet ingredients, it stimulates circulation and reduces blood pressure. Fresh, tangy orange juice marries beautifully with smooth and rich coconut milk. The juice boosts your immune system with its abundance of vitamin C. Kale's sulfur compounds clear toxins and carcinogens from your body, and fresh lime juice helps to improve digestive function and increases metabolism. All of these ingredients, when combined, showcase the magnificent interplay of sweet, tang, and spice.

Time: 5 minutes

Equipment: Blender

Yield: Approximately one 20-ounce (570 ml) smoothie

Ingredients:
1 large handful spinach
2 large kale leaves, de-ribbed and chopped
½ lime, juiced
½ small jalapeño, half of seeds removed
1 cup (235 ml) fresh orange juice
¼ cup (60 ml) coconut milk
½ cup (120 ml) coconut water

Preparation:
In a blender, combine all the ingredients.

Blend on high for 20 seconds or until smooth. Enjoy immediately and sip slowly.

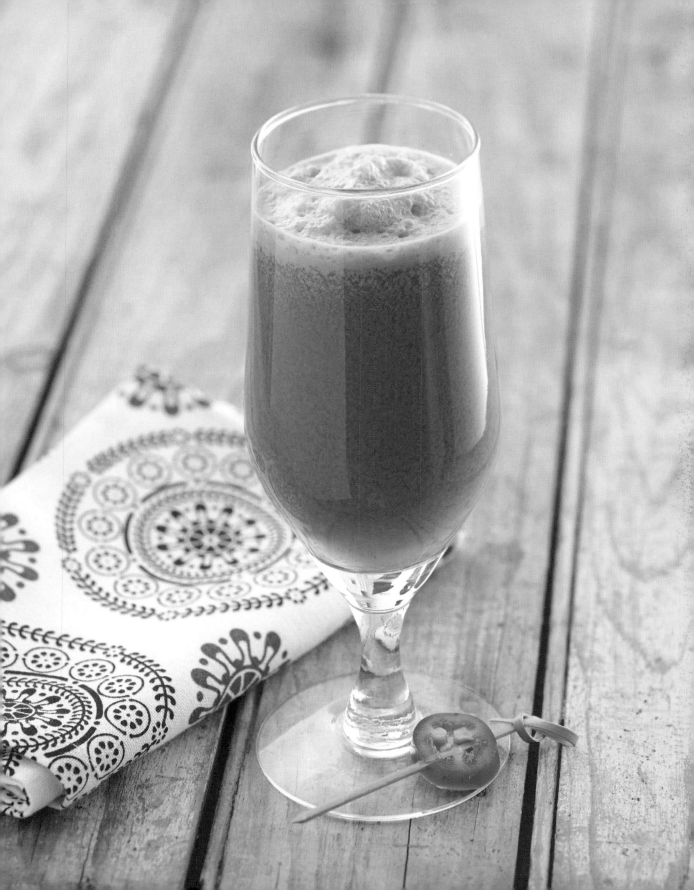

✦DREAM BAR SMOOTHIE✦

Remember dream bars? The sweet, gooey, and coconut-rich treats often included in holiday cookie tins? As a child, the tins gifted to our family would include only one or two dream bars among the tasty bunch, and my three brothers and I would fight over who would get a bite of the tantalizing treat. Today, I no longer have to elbow my way through sibling rivalry to relish in dream bar decadence. I just blend up ingredients reminiscent of the dessert, and because the ingredients are super nutritious, I don't feel the least bit guilty! This smoothie is sweetened with sugary dates, which happen to be high in fiber. The fiber staves off hunger and keeps your bowels happy. Coconut butter helps burn calories from its high percentage of medium-chain fatty acids, and coconut water not only sweetens naturally, it also hydrates. Pecans contribute to this smoothie's classic dream bar taste and are rich in plant sterols, known for their cholesterol-lowering ability.

Time: 5 minutes

Equipment: Blender

Yield: Approximately one 12-ounce (355 ml) smoothie

Ingredients:

1 tablespoon (16 g) coconut butter

4 pitted medjool dates

1 tablespoon (7 g) pecans

1 teaspoon vanilla extract

½ cup (120 ml) light coconut milk

¾ cup (177 ml) coconut water

1 teaspoon unsweetened shredded coconut

Preparation:

In a blender, combine the coconut butter, dates, pecans, vanilla, coconut milk, and coconut water.

Blend on high for 20 seconds or until smooth.

Transfer to a serving glass and sprinkle with shredded coconut. Enjoy immediately and sip slowly.

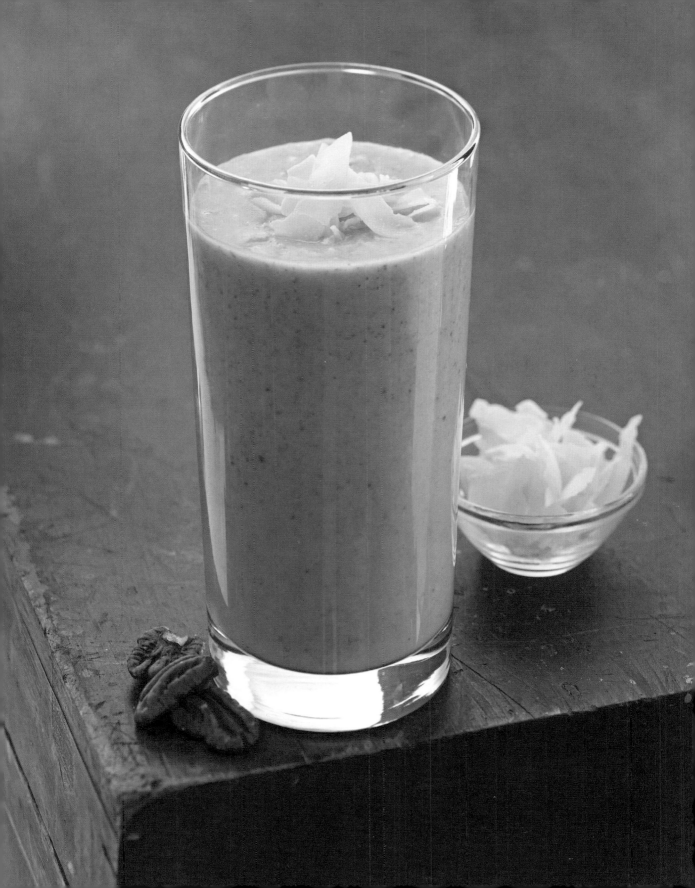

✦C2O ORANGE FRESCA✦

I have shopped so much for coconut water that instead of writing out the words on every grocery list, I just abbreviate coconut water to C2O. This refreshing tonic combines cooling C2O and fresh orange juice, resulting in a sweet and tangy beverage perfect for sipping on a hot summer day. Whole chia seeds expand in water, creating a gel-like consistency that is exceptionally good for digestion and the removal of toxins from your body. Shredded, unsweetened coconut increases your body's ability to ward off infections and the zest of an orange is abundantly rich in vitamin C, an effective immune booster and skin-toning nutrient.

Time: 25 minutes

Equipment: Small glass, blender, and large jar

Yield: Approximately one 16-ounce (475 ml) fresca

Ingredients:

2 teaspoons (5 g) chia seeds

¼ cup (60 ml) water

1 tablespoon (5 g) unsweetened shredded coconut

¼ teaspoon orange zest

¾ cup (175 ml) fresh orange juice

1 tablespoon (20 g) maple syrup

½ cup (20 ml) coconut water

10 ice cubes

Preparation:

In a small glass, combine the chia seeds and water and let rest at room temperature for ten minutes. Stir and let rest another ten minutes.

Meanwhile, in a blender, combine the shredded coconut, orange zest, orange juice, maple syrup, coconut water, and ice.

Blend on high for 20 seconds.

Transfer to a large jar and stir in the chia seeds and their soaking water. Enjoy immediately and sip slowly.

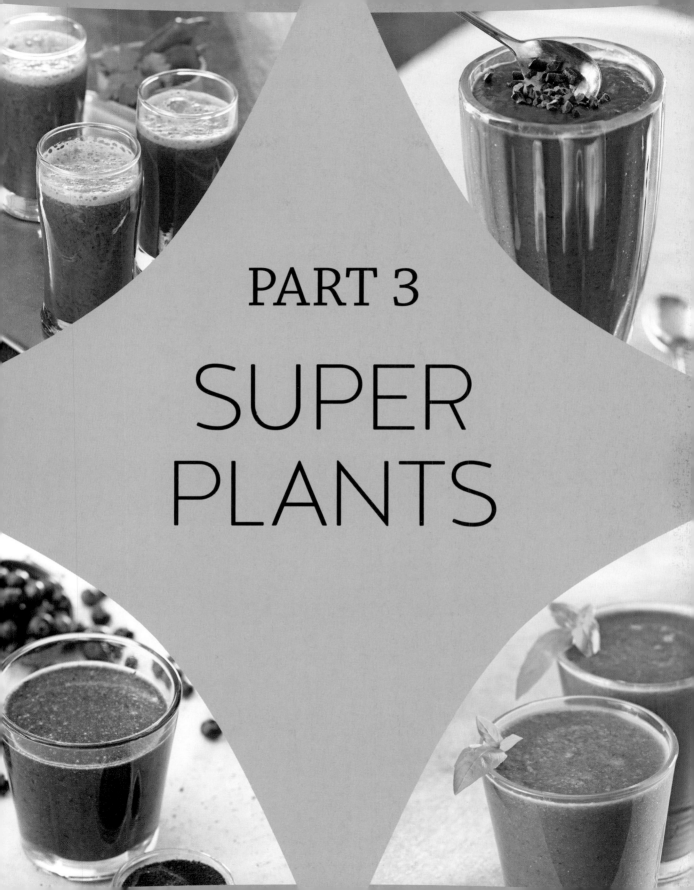

PART 3

SUPER PLANTS

CHAPTER 12

KALE

THE MEGA FLAVONOID SUPER GREEN

FEATURED RECIPES

Hot Mess Juice

Green Guru Juice

Herbalicious Smoothie

Mint Chip Smoothie

Farmacy Juice

If you have tried kale before and did not care for it, please don't give up on it just yet. If you have found the Tuscan variety to be too waxy or curly kale to be too tough on the teeth, give a different type a try. Better yet, change the way in which you eat it. You may find yourself adoring this dark leafy green if you blend it into a smoothie, marinate it with lemon juice and sea salt, or bake it into crispy kale chips.

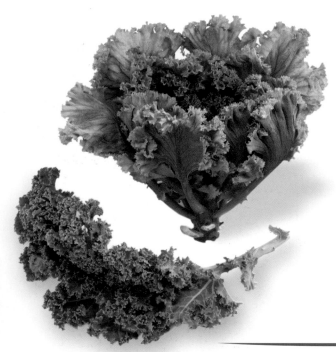

KALE: THE ULTIMATE BEAUTIFYING FOOD

Raw kale is a fantastic source of vitamins and minerals. Did you know that 1 cup (67 g) of raw kale contains only 34 calories and 90 milligrams of calcium? This is nearly 10 percent of your recommend daily value (RDV). Calcium is an essential mineral for developing and maintaining strong bones, hair, teeth, and nails. Without an adequate intake of calcium, degenerative diseases such as osteoporosis (known as porous bones) can develop, leading to an increased risk of fractures and overall bone fragility.

One cup (67 g) of raw kale also contains 80 milligrams of vitamin C, which is 134 percent of the RDV. Vitamin C is a powerful antioxidant that helps support healthy skin elasticity and boosts the immune system.

A large contributor to the aging process is oxidative stress, the burden placed on your body by exposure to environmental and food toxins. One of the easiest and most natural ways to maintain your fountain of youth is to eat an antioxidant-rich diet. Kale contains powerful antioxidants known as carotenoids and flavonoids that help to fight free radicals and slow the aging process. Free radicals can damage healthy cells and are believed to increase the risk and progression of cancer, cardiovascular disease, and age-related diseases. Adding kale to your salads, smoothies, and juices is an excellent way to ensure you get the youthful glow of radiant health!

LADIES, YOU ARE GOING TO LOVE KALE

According to Amy Scholten, MPH, at Harvard Medical School, a low dietary intake of essential vitamins and minerals can increase premenstrual syndrome (PMS) symptoms. Those that help reduce PMS symptoms, she says, include calcium, magnesium, manganese, zinc, and vitamins E and D. Does kale contain these PMS-fighting nutrients? You better believe it. In abundant quantities!

Do you experience constipation, bloating, or acne breakouts during your period? A fibrous diet, which includes foods like kale, can improve bowel regularity and lessen bloating. To combat breakouts, fuel your body with detoxifying and antioxidant-rich kale as it rids the body of environmental and dietary toxins that contribute to acne.

CRUCIFEROUS KALE FIGHTS CANCER

Kale is a member of the cruciferous family, which is known for its antioxidant and cancer-fighting properties. According to the American Cancer Society, "Cancer remains the second most common cause of death in the United States." In an article published on their site in January 2013, they noted that nearly 575,000 Americans die each year from cancer and that nearly one-third of the deaths are related to lack of exercise, poor nutrition, and obesity and thus can be prevented. This is where kale comes to the rescue. Not only is it low in calories, it is also full of fiber and essential nutrients that support long-term health.

The Chinese Cancer Prevention Study published in 1993 was one of the first large randomized trial on antioxidants and the risk of cancer. This trial investigated the effect of a combination of vitamin E, beta-carotene, and selenium on cancer. Researchers tested these nutrients on Chinese men and women at high risk for gastric cancer. The study demonstrated that when combined, these three nutrients reduced their subjects' risk of gastric and other cancers.

We can't talk about kale without giving credit to it as a fantastic source of flavonoids. There are more than forty-five varieties of flavonoids, such as kaempferol and quercetin, in kale, which have been shown to reduce allergy symptoms in test tube and animal studies. Flavonoids provide both antioxidant and anti-inflammatory benefits, making kale a leading super green for reducing chronic inflammation and oxidative stress.

Sourcing and Care of Kale

Kale is in season and available year round. To maintain lasting freshness, store in the refrigerator and wash only when ready to eat. If you wash kale too soon, it will become limp. The dark leafy green can last up to seven days if stored properly.

To prepare, first wash and dry thoroughly. Then "zip" the leaves off of the rib. To do this, take hold of the base of its rigid rib with one hand and then grab ahold of the leaves with the other. Gently pull the leaves off of the rib in the opposite direction. Compost the rib or pass it through your juicer. Enjoy the leaves in salads, smoothies, and soups or baked into kale chips.

✦HOT MESS JUICE✦

We all know what a "hot mess" is: a person who is well put together in style and appearance but who can get a little fiery and hot-headed when they've had a little too much of a good time. Well, this juice is like that late night diva in disarray. On the surface, its flavors are well constructed, compatible, and attractive, but you are caught off guard by the touch of heat and zest that comes out to play in your mouth. You'll be sure to say, "Wow, I wasn't expecting that!" But nonetheless, you'll love it anyway.

Cilantro is not an herb we often see in juicy delights, but it works wonders in this blend both nutritionally and in taste. It is one of the richest plant sources of vitamin K, supporting the health and strength of your bones, and its flavor is one of citrus and sage, which harmonize with orange and apple. Spinach provides a megadose of phytochemicals that detoxify and nourish your cells, and the gem responsible for adding a bit of fire to the mix is the jalapeño. It boosts your metabolism, burns calories, and increases circulation. Ready? Let's party!

Time: 5 minutes

Equipment: Juicer

Yield: Approximately one 16-ounce (475 ml) juice

Ingredients:

1 small handful fresh cilantro

½ jalapeño, seeds removed

2 cups (60 g) spinach

2 large kale leaves

4 large romaine leaves

1½ oranges, peeled with pith intact

1½ medium sweet apples (such as Red Delicious), halved

Preparation:

Pass the cilantro, jalapeño, spinach, kale, romaine, oranges, and apple through a juicer in the order specified.

Transfer to a large serving glass or jar. Enjoy immediately and sip slowly.

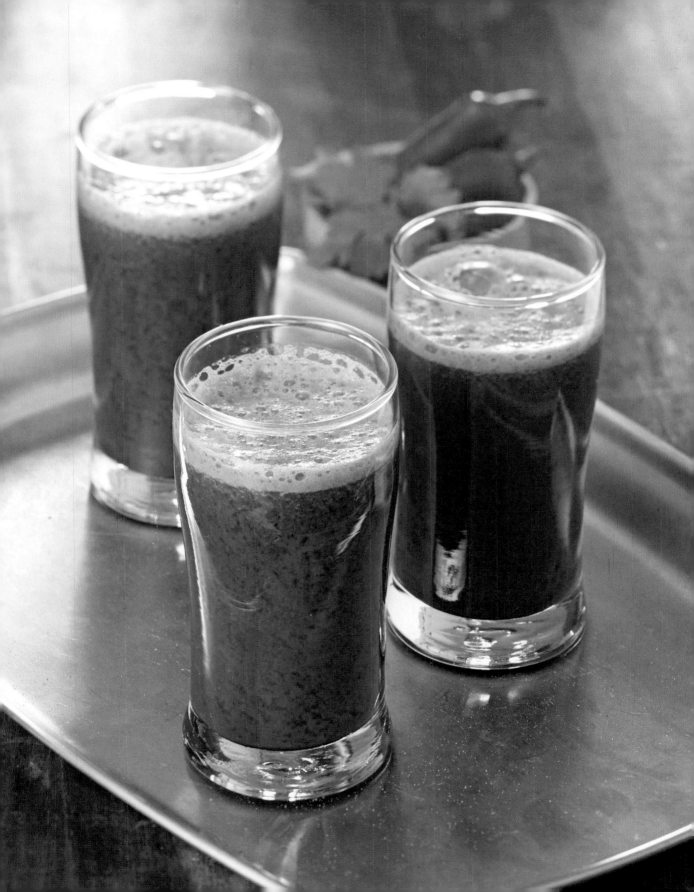

✦GREEN GURU JUICE✦

Drinking this juice will give you bragging rights for how many greens you can sip in a day. Popeye won't even be able to compete. Two cups (60 g) of spinach give you 20 percent of your daily requirement of calcium, and tart green apples keep the doctor away by delivering a healthy dose of gut-friendly bacteria. This boost of microflora increases your immunity and protects you from digestive disorders. Romaine, believe it or not, is full of nutrients such as folate, which increases your energy levels and regulates mood. Cucumber hydrates, brightens your complexion, and is a natural hormone balancer, and a touch of sea salt not only enhances the flavor of this green tonic, it provides magnesium and potassium, two essential minerals. This juice is fresh and vibrant and will make your mouth pucker with its strong tart flavor as the green apples take center stage.

Time: 5 minutes

Equipment: Juicer

Yield: Approximately one 16-ounce (475 ml) juice

Ingredients:
1 small handful parsley
2 cups (60 g) of spinach
2 large kale leaves
4 large romaine leaves
4 celery stalks, ends trimmed
1 medium cucumber, ends trimmed
2 medium green apples, halved
Pinch sea salt

Preparation:
Pass the parsley, spinach, kale, romaine, celery, cucumber, and green apples through a juicer in the order specified.

Transfer to a large serving glass or jar and stir in the sea salt. Enjoy immediately and sip slowly.

✦HERBALICIOUS SMOOTHIE✦

An unexpected blend of juicy grapefruit, cilantro, parsley, sweet coconut water, and a hint of cumin are sure to make you go "Mmmm!" Not only is its flavor uniquely delicious, this herbalicious smoothie is also full of antioxidants, vitamins, and minerals that keep your body in tip-top condition. Vitamins C, A, E, and K are plentiful and support healthy tissue repair, clear skin, bright eyes, and a strong immune system. Calcium, magnesium, and potassium help your body stay hydrated, your GI tract happy, and your muscles feeling strong and nourished. Drink up!

Time: 5 minutes

Equipment: Blender

Yield: Approximately one 20-ounce (570 ml) smoothie

Ingredients:
1 small handful cilantro
1 small handful parsley
2 large kale leaves, de-ribbed
1 large handful spinach
⅛ teaspoon cumin
¾ cup (175 ml) fresh Ruby
    Red grapefruit juice
1½ cups (355 ml) coconut water

Preparation:
In a blender, combine all the ingredients.

Blend on high for 20 seconds or until smooth. Enjoy immediately and sip slowly.

✦MINT CHIP SMOOTHIE✦

One of my favorite treats as a child was mint chocolate chip ice cream. When I gave up dairy more than four years ago, I vowed not to give up enjoying those two compatible flavors. After a few rounds of testing, I landed on a healthful smoothie that captures the essence of this summertime treat. The flavor is so lip licking that you won't notice the abundance of calcium and antioxidant-rich kale or the fibrous avocado I've snuck into this recipe.

Time: 5 minutes

Equipment: Blender

Yield: Approximately one 20-ounce (570 ml) smoothie

Ingredients:

4 large kale leaves, de-ribbed

½ medium avocado

10 to 12 fresh mint leaves

2 tablespoons (15 g) chocolate plant protein powder (such as pea or hemp)

1 tablespoon (6 g) cacao powder

1½ cups (355 ml) unsweet- ened almond milk

2 tablespoons (13 g) yacon syrup

4 to 6 ice cubes

1 teaspoon cacao nibs

Preparation:

In a blender, combine the kale, avocado, mint, protein powder, cacao powder, almond milk, yacon syrup, and ice.

Blend on high for 20 seconds or until smooth.

Transfer to a serving glass or jar and sprinkle with the cacao nibs. Enjoy immediately and sip slowly.

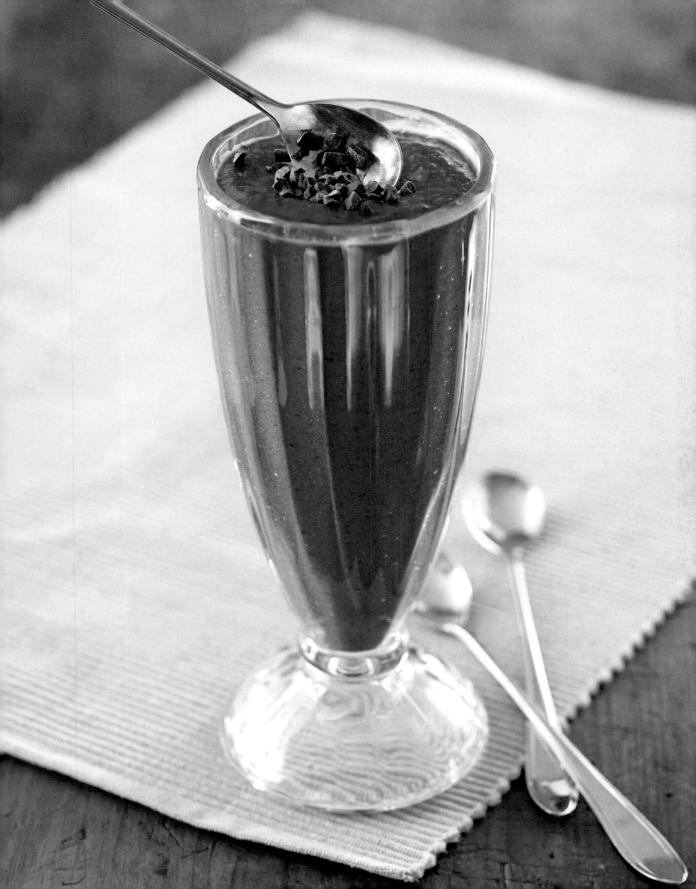

✦FARMACY JUICE✦

All of this juice's green goodness and the detoxifying power of lemon give you the natural health remedies you want for your body that you can't get in a pill from a pharmacy. The abundance of parsley, dandelion, and kale are what put the "farm" in the Farmacy Juice. With every sip, you'll feel nourished to the core as an abundance of plant-based and illness-preventing nutrients make their way through your veins. Dandelion is a powerful detoxifying and beautifying green, grapefruit is loaded with immune-boosting vitamin C, and parsley contains an abundance of antioxidants to support the health of your cells. What's most exciting is you get all this nourishment in a sweet, tangy, and succulent juice you can enjoy any time of the day.

Time: 5 minutes

Equipment: Juicer

Yield: Approximately one 16-ounce (475 ml) juice

Ingredients:

1 small handful parsley

1 small handful dandelion leaves (about 5 to 6)

1 medium lemon, peeled, with pith intact

4 large kale leaves

1½ Ruby Red grapefruits, peeled, with pith intact

Preparation:

Pass the parsley, dandelion, lemon, kale, and grapefruit through a juicer in the order specified.

Enjoy immediately and sip slowly.

SPIRULINA

NATURE'S DETOXIFIER

FEATURED RECIPES
Spicy Spirulina Juice
Salsa Verde Smoothie
Orange-a-Lina Juice
Berry Creamy Smoothie
Cold Contender Smoothie

Spirulina is blue-green algae, very similar to chlorella. It is a member of the cyanobacteria family, which thrives in warm, alkaline bodies of fresh water. It is not a new or trendy super supplement that will soon fade in popularity. In fact, spirulina dates back to the sixteenth-century Aztecs, who regularly consumed it as a food source. Spirulina is best known for its immune-boosting and detoxifying properties and for providing the body with high-quality, plant-based protein. The blue-green algae impart a taste reminiscent of roasted nori—slightly nutty with a hint of the sea. The juices and smoothies you'll soon enjoy contain ingredients that pair seamlessly with spirulina, allowing its mild seaweed flavor to settle nicely into the background.

VEGAN AND VEGETARIAN PROTEIN SOURCE

When most people think of protein sources, they visualize chicken, fish, beef, and eggs. If vegetarian or vegan, they often consider protein sources to be beans, nuts, seeds, and soy. But very few think of spirulina as a go-to source for protein intake. Spirulina is predominantly protein, between 65 and 71 percent by variety, and the protein is also complete. As noted earlier, a complete protein contains all nine essential amino acids. Just to show you how this super algae measures up to other protein sources, beef consists of only 22 percent complete protein, and the content of lentils is no more than 25 percent. Spirulina's protein abundance is staggering in comparison.

Why does this matter? Because protein is a vital macronutrient and a deficiency can lead to serious health conditions. According to the U.S. National Library of Medicine as well as the National Institutes of Health, "Every cell in the human body contains protein. It is a major building block for the skin, muscles, organs, and glands. Protein is also found in all bodily fluids, except bile and urine. You need protein in your diet to help your body repair cells and make new ones. Protein is also important for growth and development during childhood, adolescence, and pregnancy."

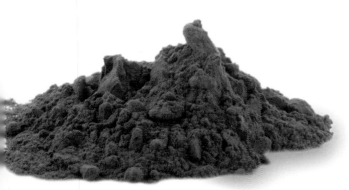

Spirulina is such a unique protein source because unlike animal proteins and ready-to-eat beans and pulses, spirulina has a longer shelf life, minimal food-safety concerns, and does not require cooking prior to consumption.

SPIRULINA FOR HEAVY METAL DETOXIFICATION

We are regularly exposed to toxins such as air pollution, heavy metals, pesticides, radiation, and other health-inhibiting substances. Over time, this level of toxicity wears on the body, resulting in illness and fatigue. It can lead to degenerative disease such as cancer and cardiovascular disease, and spirulina has a magnificent ability to bind to disease-promoting toxins and remove them.

This process of toxin elimination is known as chelation. Spirulina is a natural chelating agent, effectively binding to poisonous substances such as mercury, arsenic, and lead. The poisons are then converted to a chemically dormant form and excreted from the body without further interaction with the organs. Spirulina easily absorbs the toxins around it. Think of it like a dry sponge that when placed in water absorbs and holds onto all the water it can. Spirulina facilitates the same action with toxins in your body.

Detoxification is so important because a toxic body is at risk for serious health conditions. In addition, toxicity affects our appearance. Poor skin quality, blemishes, acne, and dry and brittle nails can all be the results of a body that is inundated with toxicity. Incorporating more plant-based foods such as spirulina into your diet helps the body rid itself of harmful substances and replenish itself with optimal nutrients to truly be healthy from the inside out.

Sourcing and Care of Spirulina

Because spirulina readily absorbs toxins, you will want to be sure to select only high-quality organic spirulina, just as you would for all your plant-based foods. Spirulina can be found in powder, tablet, capsule, and crystal forms. How much is a healthy dose? Robert Henrikson, director of the world's largest spirulina farm, states, "Typically, the Japanese, who affirm the nutrient power of spirulina, ingest 4 grams every day (equivalent to eight 500 mg tablets) and many eat even more as part of their regular program for maintaining long-term health."

It is safe to consume higher doses, but it is always best to introduce any new supplement with the lowest recommended dose and slowly increase as your body adjusts.

Store all forms of spirulina in a cool, dry, and dark environment. The algae will stay fresh up to six months once opened, although it is best to consume it within three months to achieve the maximum benefit.

✦SPICY SPIRULINA JUICE✦

Pectin, a soluble fiber, is contained in the skins of raw apples. When juiced, some of this digestion-enhancing nutrient is passed along, supporting regular and comfortable bathroom visits. Apples also deliver "good" bacteria. These microorganisms aid in the formation of healthy cells that line the intestine. Good news for you because a healthy gut is synonymous with a healthy body. Fresh ginger, the spice in this mouth-puckering juice, also supports gut health and reduces inflammation in the body. And, parsley does not only serve to liven up the flavor of this nourishing tonic, it is also rich in vitamin K, a nutrient essential to bone health.

Time: 5 minutes

Equipment: Juicer

Yield: Approximately one 16-ounce (475 ml) juice

Ingredients:
1 large handful spinach leaves

1 small handful fresh parsley

1 piece (½ inch, or 1 cm) fresh ginger

3 medium semisweet apples (such as Gala), halved

½ teaspoon spirulina crystals

Preparation:
Pass the spinach, parsley, ginger, and apples through a juicer in the order specified.

Transfer to a large serving glass or jar and stir in the spirulina crystals. Enjoy immediately and sip slowly.

✦SALSA VERDE SMOOTHIE✦

Sometimes it's nice to have a not-so-sweet smoothie. I enjoy this one nearly every day, and as a result, I feel deeply nourished and satisfied. Cucumber is cooling to the body and contains a high level of zinc, a skin-beautifying mineral. Avocado thickens the smoothie and provides hunger-fighting fiber. Fresh cilantro adds a hint of savor and blends harmoniously with alkalinizing and immune-boosting lime juice. An abundance of spinach delivers your calcium needs for the day, and spirulina crystals pack in the protein.

Time: 5 minutes

Equipment: Blender

Yield: Approximately one 20-ounce (570 ml) smoothie

Ingredients:

2 large handfuls spinach

¼ medium avocado

½ medium cucumber, ends trimmed, and chopped

2 celery stalks, ends trimmed, and chopped

1 small handful cilantro leaves

1 teaspoon spirulina crystals

½ lime, juiced

Pinch of sea salt

1½ cups (355 ml) water

Preparation:

In a blender, combine all the ingredients.

Blend on high for 20 seconds. Enjoy immediately and sip slowly.

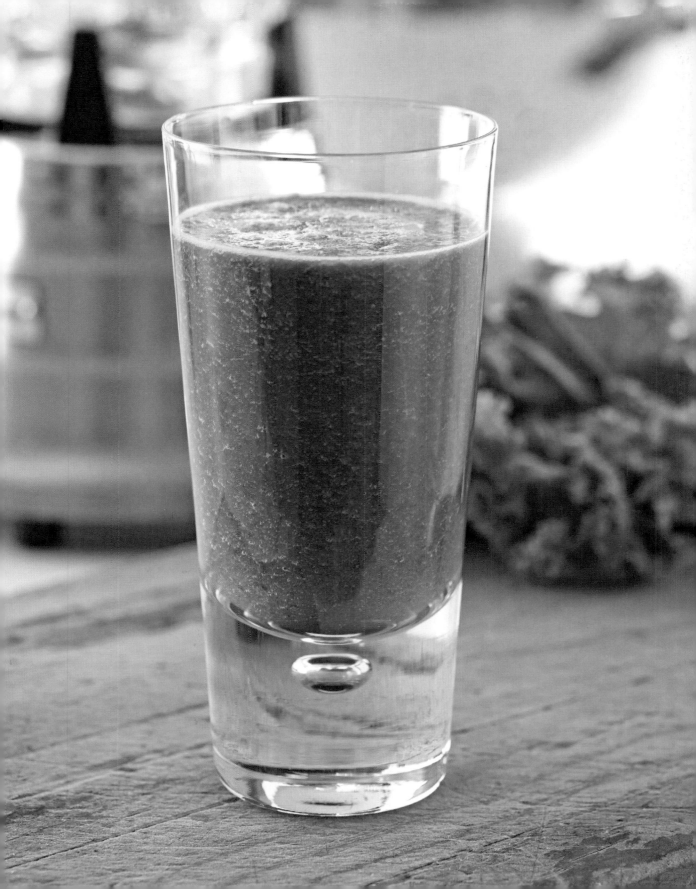

✦ORANGE-A-LINA JUICE✦

Wake up to this sweet and zingy apple-orange juice and start your day with natural and energy stimulating sugars blended with a serving of highly absorbable protein. This juice blend is simple to make, refreshing, and rich in vitamins and minerals.

Time: 5 minutes

Equipment: Juicer

Yield: Approximately one 16-ounce (455 ml) juice

Ingredients:

2 oranges, peeled, with pith in tact

1 medium tangy apple (such as a Fuji), halved

½ teaspoon spirulina crystals

Preparation:

Pass the oranges and apple through a juicer.

Transfer to a large serving glass or jar and stir in the spirulina crystals. Enjoy immediately and sip slowly.

✦BERRY CREAMY SMOOTHIE✦

Imagine a dessert of berries and cream and you have captured the essence of this dreamy smoothie. Sweetened only by the natural sugars of antioxidant-rich berries and hydrating coconut water, this recipe is a guilt-free treat. It's smooth and satisfying and has a perfect balance of fiber, protein, healthy fats, and carbohydrates. As you sip, you will feel energized, balanced, and nourished to the core.

Time: 5 minutes

Equipment: Blender

Yield: Approximately one 20-ounce (570 ml) smoothie

Ingredients:
½ cup (75 g) frozen mixed berries

1 teaspoon spirulina crystals

¼ medium avocado

1 tablespoon (5 g) unsweetened shredded coconut

1½ cups (355 ml) coconut water

Preparation:
In a blender, combine all the ingredients.

Blend on high for 20 seconds or until smooth. Enjoy immediately and sip slowly.

✦COLD CONTENDER✦ SMOOTHIE

Ward off seasonal sickness with the balanced flavors of spice and sweetness. Fibrous avocado and potassium-rich banana create this smoothie's creamy base and help you feel full and deeply nourished for hours. Spirulina aids in the detoxification of your blood, and the warming spices of cinnamon, cayenne, and ginger boost the immune system and rev your metabolism. A megadose of vitamin C is released from puréed orange and serves to protect your body during cold season.

Time: 5 minutes

Equipment: Blender

Yield: Approximately one 20-ounce (570 ml) smoothie

Ingredients:
¼ medium avocado

1 small banana, peeled

1 large naval orange, peeled, and segmented

1 teaspoon spirulina crystals

¼ teaspoon ground cinnamon

⅛ teaspoon ground cayenne

1 piece (½ inch, or 1 cm) fresh ginger, peeled

1½ cups (355 ml) coconut milk

Preparation:
In a blender, combine all the ingredients.

Blend on high for 20 seconds or until smooth. Enjoy immediately and sip slowly.

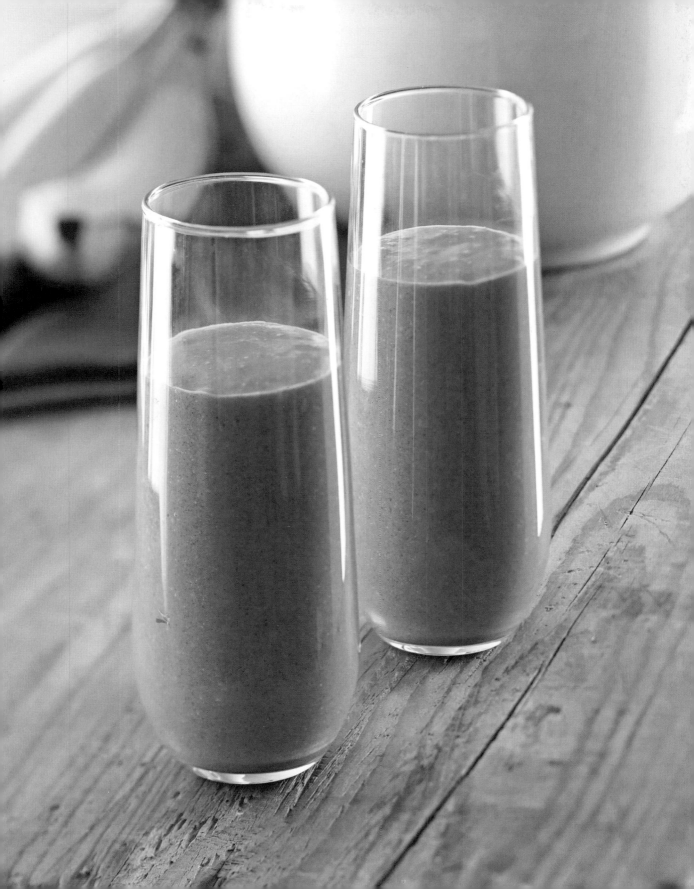

CHAPTER 14

CHLORELLA

THE VITALITY PLANT

FEATURED RECIPES

Purple Sea Monster Smoothie
Mint Apple Kiss Juice
Coconut with a Kick Smoothie
Green Tea-zer Smoothie
Sunburst Smoothie

Given the tumultuous roller coaster of everyday life, you may wonder, "Can't I just take a magic pill to make sure my body functions optimally even when I tend to overwork it?"

The answer is, "Yes!" There is a magical, nutty-tasting whole food pellet that reduces the effects of stress on your system and soothes an overworked body. It encourages cellular support and repels free radicals, those disease-promoting atoms that invade your body through stress and environmental and food toxins. This magic pill is a pressed tab, actually, the size of a pea and with the same vibrant green hue. This tiny tablet helps to restore your health with an abundance of vitalizing attributes. This wonder food is chlorella.

AN UNBREAKABLE BOND ELIMINATES TOXINS

Chlorella holds the keys to longevity, nutritive balance, and detoxification and has numerous healing properties. It is small and unassuming, yet powerful and life-affirming. Chlorella is a single-celled green algae and can be found in tablet, granulated, or powdered form. The convenient tablets allow you to take the superfood with you wherever you go; just what you need to support your busy lifestyle.

Chlorella has an unbeatable ability to neutralize and bind to nasty health inhibitors such as heavy metals, pesticides, carcinogens, and radioactive materials. This binding action helps to safely eliminate these toxins from your body and shield you from disease. For decades, the super algae have been used for this purpose throughout Asia. The Japanese rely on chlorella for its detoxifying properties and its effectiveness in binding to and removing alcohol from the liver. They also affirm its efficiency in the safe elimination of heavy metals such as cadmium and mercury and certain pesticides and herbicides from our tissues and bowels.

Clinical nutritionist Bernard Jensen, DO, PhD, said in his book, *Chlorella: Jewel of the Far East,* "I feel that chlorella's main contribution to the body's natural defense system is its beneficial supportive effects

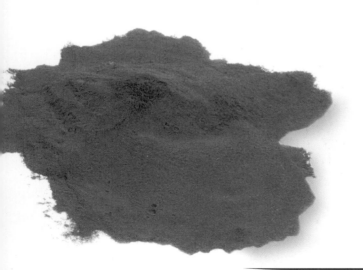

on so many of the organs and systems, especially the immune system and elimination channels. . . . The tough cellulose membrane of chlorella (which is not digested) binds to cadmium, lead, and other heavy metals and carries them out of the body."

IMMUNE-BOOSTING POWER TO BOAST ABOUT

Chlorella is also an effective immune booster because of its ability to enhance gut health. Because most of our immune system resides in our gut, healthy GI function is synonymous with immunity strength. Chlorella promotes the growth of *lactobacillus*, beneficial bacteria that contribute to a healthy colon. The green superfood aptly gets its name from chlorophyll, because it contains more of this sun-energy-dependent molecule than any other plant.

In addition, scientists have noted similarities between chlorophyll and the cell structure of our hemoglobin. It is the structure and function of chlorophyll that aid in strengthening our blood and healing disease. David Steenblock, BS, MSC, DO, in his book, *Chlorella: Natural Medicinal Algae*, said that at Kyushu University Medical College in Japan, a study was conducted on the wound-healing properties of chlorella. A group of patients who had been suffering from a variety of ailments had not recovered by way of conventional medicines, including antibiotics. They were each given chlorella as a treatment, and as a result, the wounds of three participants healed within less than three months.

PETITE-SIZED PROTEIN POWERHOUSE

It may seem untenable for algae to be rich in protein, but it is. About 60 percent of chlorella is highly absorbable protein. It contains an astonishing 15 grams in just 1 tablespoon (7 g)! That is more protein than found in most plant-based protein powders.

Sourcing and Care of Chlorella

When buying chlorella, be sure you purchase a product that is uncontaminated. In a thorough investigation and lab-controlled study conducted in 2012, a contributor to the popular health blog, Natural News, tested the cleanliness of seventeen varieties of chlorella from China, Taiwan, Japan, and Korea. He selected these regions because they are where nearly all commercially sold chlorella is sourced. The chlorella from China was the most contaminated, with Japan coming in as a close second. He discovered the cleanest varieties are from Korea and Taiwan, where the algae is grown in lab-controlled outdoor pools.

This mighty green nutrient has a shockingly long shelf life. Its nutrient power remains intact for up to eight years! For optimum freshness, store in a cool, dark, and dry environment, such as your kitchen cupboard or pantry. Most manufacturers recommend starting with a low dose and increasing as your body becomes more accustom to it. I recommend starting with 3 grams and eventually increasing to 6 grams daily.

By highly absorbable I mean that the amino acids, rather than being bound into long chains, are already broken down into smaller, more digestible chains. Many other protein sources contain long amino acid chains, which first have to be broken down in the stomach by enzymes and acid before they can be assimilated. A pretty magical, edible gem, right?

✦PURPLE SEA MONSTER✦ SMOOTHIE

Prepare to pucker up! When you sip this smoothie made with tang-tastic acai and blueberries, your taste buds are sure to be overjoyed. These two antioxidant-rich fruits add to the already incredible health profile of chlorella. This melange of superfoods boosts immunity and repels free radicals. Coconut oil stimulates metabolic function and aids in weight loss, and the medium-chain fatty acid is antibacterial, antifungal, and antiviral, aiding in the prevention of infections and disease. Sweet and refreshing coconut water is rich with electrolytes and supports hydration as do bananas due to their high level of potassium.

Time: 5 minutes

Equipment: Blender

Yield: Approximately one 20-ounce (570 ml) smoothie

Ingredients:
½ cup (75 g) blueberries

1 medium banana

2 teaspoons (9 g) coconut oil

2 teaspoons (5 g) chlorella powder

1 tablespoon (3 g) acai berry powder or ¼ cup (55 g) frozen purée

2 cups (475 ml) coconut water

Preparation:
In a blender, combine all the ingredients.

Blend on high for 20 seconds or until smooth. Enjoy immediately and sip slowly.

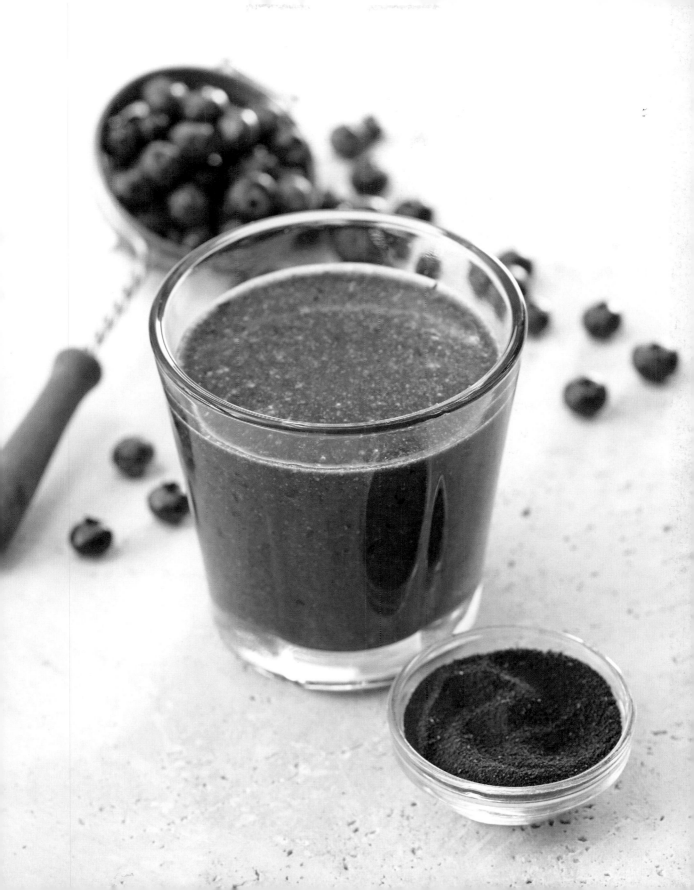

✦MINT APPLE KISS JUICE✦

Enjoy this refreshing, tart juice blend and rid your body of disease-promoting gunk. Green apples, chlorella, and mint all possess toxin-binding properties and help safely detox the body. Their three distinct flavors harmonize well and take center stage in this fresh juice blend. Your palette is first swept up in a rush of tang from the crisp apple, followed by a tinge of chlorella's nuttiness, and finished with a kiss of cooling mint. The cucumbers not only supply a cool summer day factor, but they are also high in zinc, which is an effective agent in balancing your hormones.

Time: 5 minutes

Equipment: Juicer

Yield: Approximately one 16-ounce (475 ml) juice

Ingredients:
1 large handful mint leaves
4 celery stalks, ends trimmed
1 medium cucumber, ends trimmed
2 green apples, cored, and quartered
1 teaspoon chlorella powder

Preparation:
Pass the mint, celery, cucumber, and apples through a juicer in the order specified.

Transfer to a large serving glass or jar and stir in the chlorella powder. Enjoy immediately and sip slowly.

✦COCONUT WITH A KICK✦ SMOOTHIE

Because of their shared nutty flavor, coconut and chlorella play nicely together in this creamy delight. When combined with peppery ginger, spicy cayenne, and candy-like dates, the combination of flavors is unmatched. Ginger is an excellent inflammation tamer, and the use of shredded coconut and coconut milk deliver a healthy dose of high-quality saturated fat to help keep you sated for hours.

Time: 5 minutes

Equipment: Blender

Yield: Approximately one 20-ounce (570 ml) smoothie

Ingredients:

1 handful spinach

2 large kale leaves, de-ribbed and chopped

1 tablespoon (5 g) unsweetened shredded coconut

1½ cups (355 ml) light coconut milk

4 pitted medjool dates

2 teaspoons (5 g) chlorella powder

1 teaspoon fresh ginger, grated

⅛ teaspoon cayenne pepper

Preparation:

In a blender, combine all the ingredients.

Blend on high for 20 seconds or until smooth. Enjoy immediately and sip slowly.

✦GREEN TEA-ZER SMOOTHIE✦

One of my favorite ways to enjoy antioxidant-rich yerba mate is blended into a smoothie. This tea of South American origin contains 90 percent more antioxidants than other green varieties, and though it does contain about 80 mg of caffeine per serving, its effects on the nervous system are slowed by its many other health properties. This smoothie is creamy and rich from the use of coconut milk. It is naturally sweetened with digestion enhancing yacon and plump dates, providing a flavor that is simply luscious.

Time: 5 minutes

Equipment: Blender

Yield: Approximately one 20-ounce (570 ml) smoothie

Ingredients:

1½ cups (355 ml) brewed and chilled yerba mate tea

1 teaspoon chlorella powder

½ cup (120 ml) coconut milk

3 pitted medjool dates

1 tablespoon (7 g) yacon syrup

½ teaspoon vanilla extract

Preparation:

In a blender, combine all the ingredients.

Blend on high for 20 seconds or until smooth. Enjoy immediately and sip slowly.

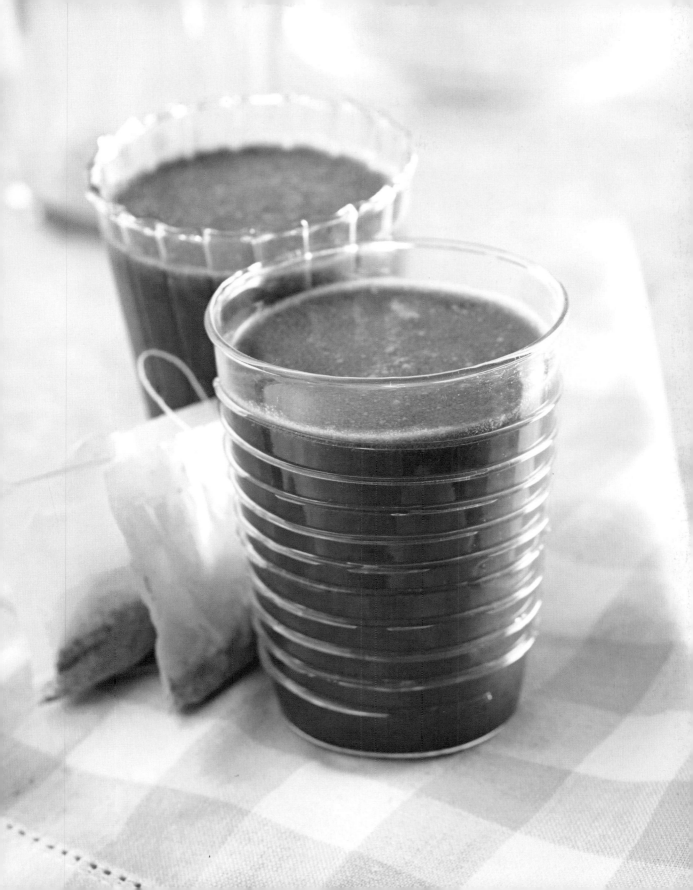

✦SUNBURST SMOOTHIE✦

Enjoy this scrumptious green smoothie perfect for an afternoon pick-me-up. Surprisingly sweet sunflower sprouts add to the abundant sugar content of pear and banana. Both integrate seamlessly with the nutty flavor of chlorella and sunflower seeds. In addition, sunflower seeds and their sprouts are rich in zinc, which supports skin clarity and elasticity. An added bonus of including sunflower sprouts is that they are 25 percent protein! With their protein punch and that of chlorella, this smoothie is so macronutrient-dense you may consider enjoying it as a meal replacement.

Time: 5 minutes

Equipment: Blender

Yield: Approximately one 20-ounce (570 ml) smoothie

Ingredients:
½ cucumber, chopped
1 large Anjou pear, cored
¼ medium banana
2 celery stalks, chopped
1 handful spinach
1 tablespoon (9 g) sunflower seeds
1 small handful sunflower sprouts
1½ teaspoons chlorella powder
1 cup (235 ml) water

Preparation:
In a blender, combine all the ingredients.

Blend on high for 20 seconds or until smooth. Enjoy immediately and sip slowly.

CHAPTER 15

WHEATGRASS

THE OXIDATIVE STRESS BUSTER

FEATURED RECIPES

Sweet Grass Juice

Latin Lover Juice

Carrot Top Juice

New Zealand Zinger Juice

Mango Grasshopper Smoothie

Wheatgrass is the inedible grass sprout of the wheat berry and can only be consumed in juice or freeze-dried powdered form. Those who swear by the superfood claim that when they consistently include wheatgrass in their health regime, they experience boosted energy, strong immunity, and a visible glow. So what makes this very popular green so enticing despite its reputation for being unpleasant tasting?

OXIDATIVE STRESS BUSTER

The first reason is oxidative stress. As described previously in this book, oxidative stress is a burden placed on our cells and tissues caused by consuming a highly acidic diet, excessive stress and anxiety, the use of tobacco, prescription drugs, and exposure to environmental pollutants. Exposure to all these toxins promotes acidity in the body, and excess acidity throws our desirable pH levels off. When our pH is not balanced and we fall into the acid zone, our risk of contracting disease increases. Why?

Bacteria, yeast, and viruses thrive in an acidic environment. Conversely, they cannot thrive in alkaline conditions. Wheatgrass, because of its nutrient-rich composition, helps to increase alkalinity and contributes to a reduction in oxidative stress and the prevention of disease. A 1995 article in the *Journal of the National Cancer Institute* stated, "Chlorophyll fed to laboratory animals reduced the absorption of three dietary carcinogens: those found in cooked meat, those from smoked and barbecued foods, and those produced by mold that infect grains and peanuts." To date, no human studies have been conducted.

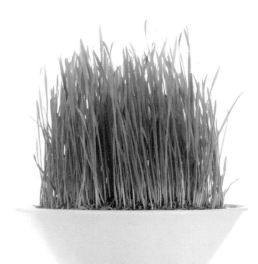

Sourcing and Care of Wheatgrass

The environment in which wheatgrass is grown determines whether it will provide you with the abundance of health benefits described previously. Much of the wheatgrass available today, including the juice available at commercial smoothie and juice bars, comes from nonorganic sprouts grown in soil void of minerals, resulting in a tonic that is nutrient deficient. It is important then to ensure that the wheatgrass you are consuming is grown locally and is 100 percent certified organic.

In addition, wheatgrass is best consumed within seven days of it sprouting. Unfortunately, you can't be sure how long it has been sitting at the juice bar or how long it was in transit before it arrived. Thus, the best way to consume wheatgrass is to sprout and juice it in your home or to purchase frozen juice cubes or freeze-dried powder. If purchasing the powder, only buy brands that clearly state the wheatgrass was harvested when the shoots were still tender and at their peak of nutrient potency. Make sure the facility processing the powder does so by first masticating the juice and then drying it at very low temperatures, no higher than 35°F (1.7°C). This helps to maintain enzyme potency. Powdered wheatgrass should be stored in your refrigerator and used within thirty days of opening.

PROVOCATIVE NUTRIENTS BEAUTIFY AND ENERGIZE

In addition to ample levels of chlorophyll, wheatgrass also contains all the B vitamins, as well as vitamins A, C, E, and K. It also has high levels of calcium, magnesium, iron, and zinc. Of the three hundred bodily functions it supports, magnesium aids in restful sleep, muscle and tissue repair, and bowel health. Zinc supports hormone regulation and reduces inflammatory skin conditions, including acne. Vitamin A is a body beautifier; it clarifies the skin, brightens the eyes, and strengthens hair and nails. Calcium, vitamin K, and magnesium all support bone growth and strength; B vitamins calm the nervous system, are essential for fat, carbohydrate, and protein synthesis, provide energy, and regulate hormone and metabolic function. Last but not least, vitamin C boosts the immune system and supports muscle and tissue health. If one shot of wheatgrass can provide all those nutrients, I certainly am going to include it in my eating routine! How about you?

✦SWEET GRASS JUICE✦

Succulent pear, cool cucumber, and fresh romaine sweeten and cut through the grassiness often associated with drinking pure wheatgrass juice. And pears don't only taste divine, they are also one of the highest known fruit sources of antioxidant-rich flavonoids. These phytonutrients protect against disease and have antiaging qualities. Cucumbers contain an abundance of the mineral zinc, which is excellent for skin and tissue health. They are also a natural diuretic, aiding in the release of toxins from the body. Romaine is rich in folate, which supports energy and mood regulation. And spinach contains magnesium, calcium, and vitamin K, all essential nutrients for the health and strength of your bones. Pretty sweet, eh?

Time: 10 minutes

Equipment: Juicer

Yield: Approximately one 16-ounce (475 ml) juice

Ingredients:
2 large handfuls spinach
4 large romaine leaves
1 cucumber, ends trimmed
2 medium pears, halved
½ teaspoon wheatgrass powder

Preparation:
Pass the spinach, romaine, cucumber, and pears through a juicer in the order specified.

Transfer to a serving glass and stir in the wheatgrass powder. Enjoy!

✦LATIN LOVER JUICE✦

This juice is definitely for the green juice guru. It is low in sugar and imparts a savory flavor from a hint of lime and touch of spice. A pinch of sea salt draws the flavors together in a taste reminiscent of green gazpacho. You can't beat the nutrient profile of this blend, and if you find you enjoy a fruitless juice, you may want to incorporate this tonic into your diet multiple times per week. Kale is rich in sulfur, a multitasking nutrient that clears toxins and carcinogens from the body, supports muscle repair, stimulates circulation, and promotes the growth of healthy gut bacteria. Jalapeño also increases circulation, lowers blood pressure, and increases metabolic burn. Parsley contains powerful antioxidants that reduce oxidative stress of the cells, and lime is antibacterial, increasing your resistance to infections. This is a powerful tonic made to heal!

Time: 10 minutes

Equipment: Juicer

Yield: Approximately one 16-ounce (475 ml) juice

Ingredients:
½ medium jalapeño, seeds optional (depending on your heat preference)
3 large handfuls spinach
1 large handful parsley
2 medium limes, skin cut away, with pith intact
4 large kale leaves
1 medium bunch romaine leaves
1 medium cucumber, ends trimmed
2 cubes frozen wheatgrass juice
Pinch sea salt

Preparation:
Pass the jalapeño, spinach, parsley, lime, kale, romaine, and cucumber through a juicer in the order specified.

Transfer to a serving glass, add the frozen wheatgrass cubes, and dissolve them in the juice. Sprinkle in sea salt and enjoy!

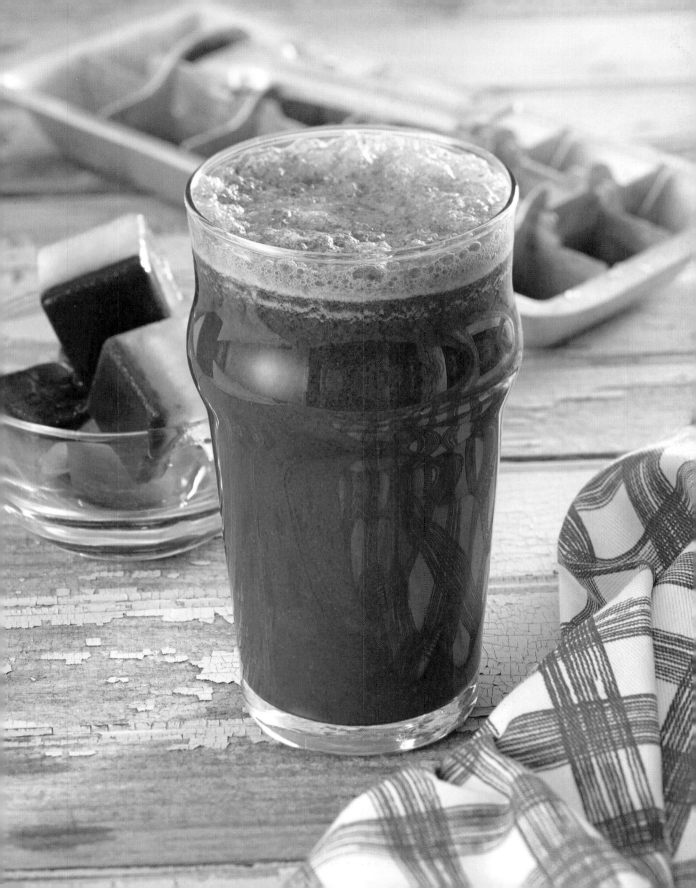

✦CARROT TOP JUICE✦

If the flavor of the wheatgrass juice has turned your nose up in the past, give it another chance. This sweet and tangy concoction is sure to have you drinking wheatgrass like a pro. Sugary carrot juice tames wheatgrass's, well, grassy taste, while beautifying your body from a boost of vitamin A. Tangy Ruby Red grapefruit and lemon add zest to the juice blend and mellow the notorious wheatgrass bite. They also deliver an abundance of vitamin C, boosting your immune system and giving your muscles and tissues a healthy dose of repair. Finally, fresh ginger adds a touch of spice, is good for your gut, and reduces inflammation.

Time: 10 minutes

Equipment: Juicer

Yield: Approximately one 16-ounce (475 ml) juice

Ingredients:

1 piece (½ inch, or 1 cm) fresh ginger

1 medium lemon, peeled, with pith intact

1 large Ruby Red grapefruit, peeled, with pith intact, and quartered

5 large carrots, ends trimmed

2 cubes frozen wheatgrass juice

Preparation:

Pass the ginger, lemon, grapefruit, and carrots through a juicer in the order specified.

Transfer to a serving glass, dissolve the wheatgrass cubes in the juice, stir, and enjoy.

✦NEW ZEALAND ZINGER✦ JUICE

With a built-in balance of tangy and sweet flavor, kiwi is an especially delicious fruit and should get more attention for its health benefits. It contains actinidin, a protein-dissolving enzyme that aids in digestion. It also contains high levels of potassium that support the balance of your electrolytes as well as an abundance of vitamin C, which boosts the immune system and slows the aging of skin. The combination of sugary-tart kiwi with tangy lemon juice and peppery ginger calms the intense flavor of wheatgrass in this exquisite juice blend.

Time: 10 minutes

Equipment: Juicer

Yield: Approximately one 16-ounce (475 ml) juice

Ingredients:
1 piece (½ inch, or 1 cm) fresh ginger
1 medium lemon, peeled, with pith intact
3 kiwis, skin cut away
1 medium cucumber, ends trimmed
2 cubes frozen wheatgrass juice

Preparation:
Pass the ginger, lemon, kiwi, and cucumber through a juicer in the order specified.

Transfer to a serving glass, dissolve the wheatgrass cubes in the juice, stir, and sip away!

✦MANGO GRASSHOPPER✦ SMOOTHIE

You can't go wrong with the tropical flavors of mango and pineapple if you want to mask the intense flavor of wheatgrass. Not to mention both pineapple and mango contain digestive enzymes that help to break down proteins for more efficient assimilation and absorption. Apple is rich in fiber and keeps your digestive system in tip-top shape. So if you're feeling like your digestion needs a little oomph, this smoothie has your name written all over it!

Time: 10 minutes

Equipment: Blender

Yield: Approximately one 20-ounce (570 ml) smoothie

Ingredients:

½ cup (90 g) fresh or frozen mango

½ teaspoon wheatgrass powder

1 large handful spinach leaves

2 large kale leaves, de-ribbed

1 medium semisweet apple (such as Fuji or Gala), cored, and quartered

1½ cups (355 ml) fresh pineapple juice

5 to 6 ice cubes

Preparation:

In a blender, combine all the ingredients.

Blend on high for 20 seconds. Enjoy immediately and say, "Ah!"

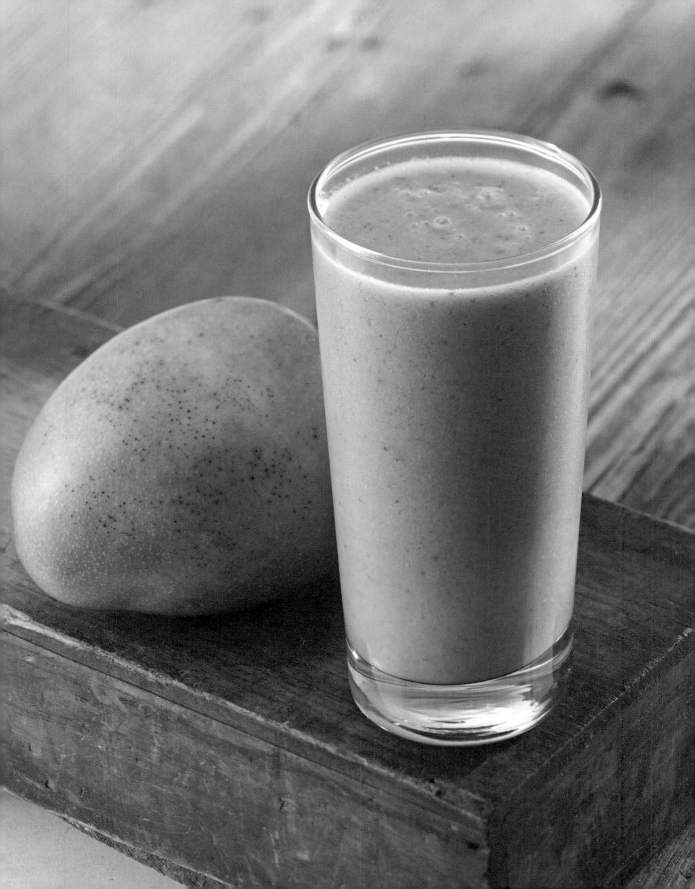

CHAPTER 16

AFA

BLUE-GREEN ALGAE: THE IMMUNE-BOOSTING ENERGIZER

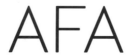

FEATURED RECIPES
The Green Mile Smoothie
The Loch Ness Juice
Apples and Algae Juice
Sweet Basil Smoothie
Watermelon Salsa Smoothie

Aphanizomenon flos-aquae (AFA) is a living water plant of the Cyanophyta family. Cyanophyta organisms grow in nearly all droplets of sunlit water, and you may know of them by their more common nomenclature, blue-green algae. Blue-green algae are among nature's most beneficial superfoods. Devout consumers of this lake-living and life-affirming food think so highly of it that they sometimes refer to it as the invisible flower of the water.

According to the Hippocrates Health Institute, Cyanophyta, which are single-cell organisms, are responsible for manufacturing 90 percent of the earth's oxygen and 80 percent of its food supply. There are nearly 1,500 species of these organisms,

with AFA being the most adored. The AFA fit for our consumption is grown in unpolluted and pristine bodies of water around the globe. These untouched and nutrient-rich environments promote ample growth of this highly nutritious life form.

ENHANCE YOUR IMMUNITY WITH AFA

In a 2000 article titled *Consumption of Aphanizomenon flos-aquae Has Rapid Effects on the Circulation and Function of Immune Cells in Humans,* six researchers at McGill University in Montreal examined the effects consumption of AFA had on the immune system. During their evaluation, they discovered AFA led to rapid changes in immune cell delivery but did not facilitate activation of lymphocytes (white blood cells). This means it boosts strength in immunity without causing an adverse immune attack.

In addition, during a study conducted at the Royal Victoria Hospital in Montreal, a research group led by Gitte S. Jensen, MD, discovered that eating AFA had a profound effect on natural killer (NK) cells. NK cells have the ability to scavenge for and recognize cancerous, diseased, or virus-infected cells and kill them, leaving healthy cells unaffected.

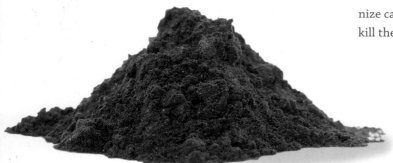

ENERGIZE WITH AFA

AFA is one of a few plant food sources that delivers an adequate amount of bioavailable vitamin B12. This vitamin is essential for the health of your nervous system, adrenal function, and energy. A deficiency can be recognized by symptoms of fatigue, muscle aches, nervousness, anxiety, brain fog, diarrhea, and even anemia (iron deficiency).

How much do you need? The US recommended daily allowance (RDA) of B12 is 2.4 mcg. One serving (1 liquid g) of AFA delivers 8 mcg! That is four times the daily recommended amount! That said, when starting out with the food supplement, it is advised by manufacturers and users to begin slowly to avoid any unpleasant side effects that can result from AFA's detoxifying qualities. They suggest beginning with only 1 teaspoon per day for about a week and then increasing to the suggested serving of 1 table-spoon (15 ml) per day. You can always take more if you need an extra energy boost. It is also recom-mended that you drink plenty of water throughout the day (at least half your weight in ounces) to flush out toxins that will be released by the natural cleansing effects of the algae.

Because vitamin B12 is found predominantly in animal protein, it is not uncommon for devout vegans and vegetarians to be deficient in this essential nutrient. If you follow a plant-based diet and feel sluggish, weak, or even a little blue, see whether a daily serving of AFA added to your morning smoothie will add a little pep back to your step.

Other plant sources of vitamin B12 are spirulina, which is similar in taste and its energizing properties, and nutritional yeast, an inactive yeast frequently used in non-dairy cheese recipes, sauces, and dress-ings for its notable and pungent cheese-like flavor. You can often find powdered spirulina and nutri-tional yeast in health food markets and online.

Sourcing and Care of AFA

AFA can be purchased from the frozen food section of most health markets or online from a variety of retailers. It should be kept frozen, thawing no more than seven servings (seven days' worth) at a time in the refrigerator. Once thawed, it must be kept cold at all times to maintain maximum nutrient potency and should be consumed within seven days per manufacturer's recommendations. Also, be sure to look for 100 percent organic and wild-harvested varieties to ensure you are consuming high-quality AFA.

✦THE GREEN MILE✦ SMOOTHIE

If you are looking for a single smoothie that delivers all the nutrients you need, look no further than this mighty delicious green juice. Vitamin- and mineral-rich kale and spinach are combined with fibrous banana, enzyme-loaded pineapple, vitamin B12-bearing AFA, and hydration-balancing coconut water. This vibrant mix of sweet and tart fruits takes the "green" taste out of this recommended daily blend.

Time: 5 minutes

Equipment: Blender

Yield: Approximately one 20-ounce (570 ml) smoothie

Ingredients:
2 handfuls spinach
4 medium kale leaves, de-ribbed
1 small banana
½ semisweet apple (such as Fuji or Gala)
½ cup (120 ml) fresh pineapple juice
1 cup (235 ml) coconut water
1 tablespoon (15 ml) AFA
4 to 5 ice cubes

Preparation:
In a blender, combine all the ingredients.

Blend on high for 20 seconds. Enjoy!

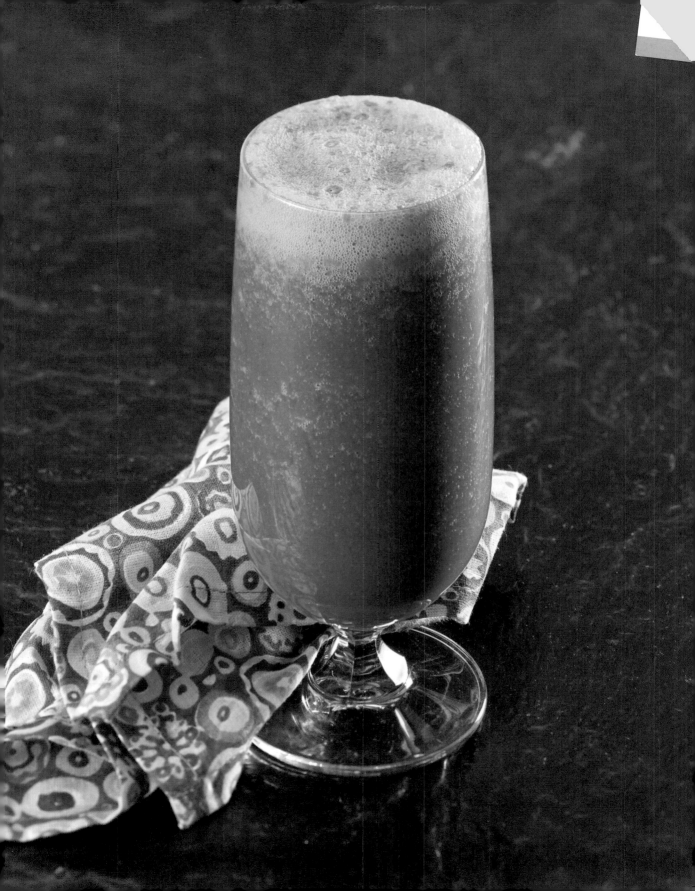

✦THE LOCH NESS JUICE✦

Sugary red grapes and tangy-sweet Ruby Red grapefruit help mask the distinct Loch Ness swamp-like taste of AFA. In addition, the grapes have antibacterial, antifungal, and antiviral properties, which help to keep illness and infections at bay. Grapefruit has a staggeringly high percentage of vitamin C, which keeps colds away, tones and beautifies the skin, and detoxifies the liver, and cucumber adds a refreshing and cooling element to the juice and contains bone-strengthening vitamin K. This joyous blend of flavors mellow AFA, making this an excellent tonic for regular algae consumption.

Time: 10 minutes

Equipment: Juicer

Yield: Approximately one 16-ounce (475 ml) juice

Ingredients:

2 large handfuls red seedless grapes

1 medium Ruby Red grapefruit, peeled, with pith intact, and quartered

5 large romaine leaves

1 medium cucumber, ends trimmed

1 tablespoon (15 ml) AFA

Preparation:

Pass the grapes, grapefruit, romaine, and cucumber through a juicer in the order specified.

Transfer to a serving glass, stir in the AFA, and enjoy!

✦APPLES AND ALGAE JUICE✦

Like peas and carrots, the fusion of apples and algae is truly harmonious. Not only do the flavors meld magnificently on their own, but when combined with cooling mint leaves, they impart a taste that is divinely refreshing. Apples are full of digestion-supporting enzymes, and when your gut is healthy, you absorb nutrients more efficiently, eliminate toxins better, and are less susceptible to disease. Celery serves as a natural diuretic to help carry waste and toxins out of the body, and it contains potassium and sodium, which support healthy tissues. I'd say drinking this tonic each day is a sure way to keep the doctor away!

Time: 5 minutes

Equipment: Juicer

Yield: Approximately one 16-ounce (475 ml) juice

Ingredients:

1 large handful fresh mint leaves

4 medium celery stalks

3 medium semisweet apples (such as Fuji or Gala), halved

1 tablespoon (15 ml) AFA

Preparation:

Pass the mint leaves, celery, and apples through a juicer.

Transfer to a serving glass, stir in the AFA, and enjoy!

✦SWEET BASIL SMOOTHIE✦

Have you ever been exposed to the incredible flavor combination of strawberries and basil? This lesser known union is to die for delicious and antioxidant-rich. Strawberries contain anthocyanins, powerful heart-healthy phytonutrients that helps drive your LDL, or bad, cholesterol down. Basil calms the nervous system and supports liver detoxification, and AFA aids in the transport of released toxins out of the body. This tasty herb-and-berry blend when met with refreshing coconut water and creamy avocado may leave you feeling like you've just died and gone to heaven.

Time: 5 minutes

Equipment: Blender

Yield: Approximately one 20-ounce (570 ml) smoothie

Ingredients:
8 fresh or frozen strawberries
1 tablespoon (15 ml) AFA
¼ medium avocado
8 basil leaves
1 handful spinach
2 cups (475 ml) coconut water

Preparation:
In a blender, combine all the ingredients.

Blend on high for 20 seconds. Enjoy immediately and sip slowly.

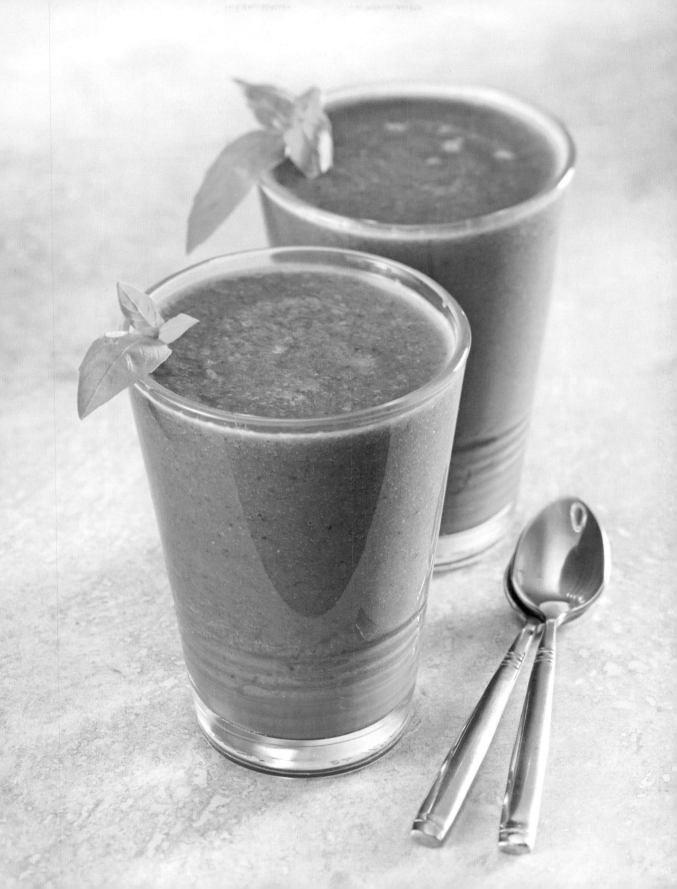

✦WATERMELON SALSA✦ SMOOTHIE

I am a total herb lover and put them in just about everything from sweet desserts to refreshing beverages, crisp salads, and many of my smoothie creations. This recipe has two magnificent herbs, mint and cilantro, that are particularly fond of mingling with sweet watermelon and tangy lime. The cooling properties of both the melon and the mint make this a nourishing summertime tonic, and lime juice helps to carry away toxins that may have accumulated from one too many barbecues. Add in sugary dates as well as creamy coconut milk and you've got a fiesta of flavor!

Time: 10 minutes

Equipment: Blender

Yield: Approximately one 20-ounce (570 ml) smoothie

Ingredients:
1 cup (150 g) fresh seedless watermelon flesh, chopped

3 pitted medjool dates

1 cup (235 ml) coconut milk

1 lime, juiced

1 tablespoon (15 ml) AFA

8 mint leaves

1 tablespoon (1 g) cilantro leaves

Preparation:
In a blender, combine all the ingredients.

Blend on high for 20 seconds. Enjoy immediately and sip slowly.

CHAPTER 17

MACA

THE PERUVIAN SUPER PLANT

FEATURED RECIPES

Fall Holiday Smoothie

Anti-Flame Yam Milk

Mexi Milk Steamer

Lover Smoothie

Lemon Rosemary Froth

Maca, also known as nature's Viagra and Peruvian ginseng among its fans, is a plant that grows in central Peru, high in the Andes Mountains, and has been cultivated there for at least three thousand years. It is a root vegetable and a relative of the spicy radish (in the cruciferous family of plants), although it tastes more like butterscotch or malt, depending on the variety.

There are multiple types of maca, with the most common being yellow, black, and red. Though they all support energy stimulation and endocrine system regulation, the results achieved by each vary from person to person.

MACA: APHRODISIAC AND ADAPTOGEN

Adaptogens are plants that de-stress and restore normal physiological functioning in the body without specific attention to any one system or organ. Adaptogens are nontoxic, contribute to whole-body balancing, and naturally increase resistance to disease. For example, if your body is producing too much of a particular hormone, the adaptogen—in this case maca—will help your body produce less of it. If your body is producing too little of a hormone, maca will kick in to help increase the amount being produced while at the same time balance all other systems to support the one out of whack.

What's really nifty is that adaptogen supplements, if needed, can be used for long periods of time without having a negative effect on any bodily function. That said, when supplementing, it is still a good idea to adjust adaptogen dosage throughout use to gain maximum benefit, but I'll cover that in a moment after I talk about something much more interesting: its sexual enhancement qualities.

Maca is most revered for its libido-enhancing and endocrine-balancing abilities. Maca nourishes and supports adrenal glands and the thyroid to produce hormones in the proper balance needed by each individual. Maca has been used to regulate mood, reduce premenstrual and menopausal symptoms, and increase sexual desire. In the 2008 edition of *CNS Neuroscience and Therapeutics*, researchers evaluated sixteen participants who were experiencing sexual dysfunction due to the use of antidepressants. After taking

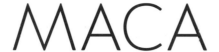

a controlled dosage of maca root as a supplement, the majority of volunteers experienced a considerable increase in sex drive.

During a twelve-week trial, men ages twenty-one to fifty-six were administered maca in either 1500 mg or 3000 mg dosages. They were evaluated at four, eight, and twelve week intervals. An improvement in sexual desire was documented at the eight-week mark without any change in testosterone and estradiol (a sex hormone) levels. This demonstrated that maca on its own can support an increase in libido.

Gary P. Gordon, MD, former president of the American College for Advancement in Medicine, was quoted on Nuturodoc.com touting his personal appreciation of maca and how he sees it benefit those he treats. Gordon said, "We all hear rumors about various products like maca. But using this Peruvian root myself, I personally experienced a significant improvement in erectile tissue response. I call it 'nature's answer to Viagra.'"

FEEL ALERT AND ACTIVE WITH MACA ROOT

Maca energizes and builds endurance because of its naturally occurring high concentration of B vitamins (your energy boosters and nervous system nutrients) and being rich in complex carbohydrates, about 60 percent. In addition, because it works to regulate the endocrine and adrenal systems, this contributes to more restful sleep, alertness, and boosts in energy.

HOW MUCH TO TAKE?

Maca manufacturers and holistic health practitioners suggest starting out with a small dose of maca and building up to no more than 1 tablespoon (15 g) per day. A good amount to start with is 1 teaspoon of the powder (equivalent to about 1500 mg). See how you feel at this level after three or four days. If feeling pleasantly alert and well, you can stay at that amount or perhaps increase by half or a full teaspoon until

Sourcing and Care of Maca

When you head out to purchase maca, buy only raw and 100 percent organic powder varieties. It can taste unpleasant if eaten alone and is best enjoyed with food. The flavors most complementary to maca are malt, the smokiness of chilies, the nutty flavor achieved from flax, coconut, almond, and hemp, the robustness of chocolate, coffee, and molasses, or the sweetness of lucuma, yacon, date, or even banana.

Maca powder can usually be found in the bulk herb section of your health food store as well as in the natural supplement aisle. Alternatively, you can purchase maca powder through multiple online retailers. Maca has a shelf life of about seven years if unopened. It does not need to be refrigerated but should be stored in a cool, dry environment. Once opened, use within one year to ensure maximum potency of micronutrients.

you reach a maximum of 1 tablespoon (15 g). Because maca also has energy-boosting qualities, some who take the supplement can feel jittery or excessively energized if they take too much and may need to cut the dosage in half. Also, for this same reason, it is best to take maca in the morning as doing so in the evening can disrupt sleep.

For every week you take the supplement, it is a good idea to take a day off and for every full month of usage, step back from use for one week. As with all food supplements, whenever you have reached the desired effects, it is best to stop taking the supplement and only reintroduce as needed.

✦FALL HOLIDAY SMOOTHIE✦

Get your sweats on and get cozy because this smoothie is going to take you straight to holiday season. It's such a delicious way to use antioxidant- and fiber-rich pumpkin purée. Now you can enjoy the warm spice and creamy sweet flavors of pumpkin pie without all the junk that you don't need. Coconut butter adds a layer of complexity that imparts a touch of nuttiness, while revving your metabolism with its abundance of medium-chain fatty acids, and the rich spices of clove and cinnamon naturally increase circulation, warming you from the inside out!

Time: 5 minutes

Equipment: Blender

Yield: Approximately one 20-ounce (570 ml) smoothie

Ingredients:
¾ cup (184 g) pumpkin purée

¼ medium avocado

1½ cups (355 ml) unsweet-
  ened almond milk

2 tablespoons (32 g) coconut butter

2 teaspoons (10 g) maca powder

2 tablespoons (13 g) yacon
  or (40 g) maple syrup

1 teaspoon vanilla extract

½ teaspoon ground cinnamon

⅛ teaspoon ground cloves

Pinch sea salt

Pinch allspice

Preparation:
In a blender, combine all the ingredients.

Blend on high for 20 seconds or until smooth. Sip and savor!

+ANTI-FLAME YAM MILK+

Oh my goodness, I love this milky blend so much! Not only does it taste amazing, it is antioxidant-rich, anti-inflammatory, libido-boosting, energizing, and digestion enhancing as well! How's that for a nourishment lineup? Turmeric and yam are the responsible parties for driving down inflammation. Maca tends to get your libido rocking, dates sweeten and energize, and all of the warm spices support digestive health and increase circulation and metabolism. The flavor of this creamy delight is an incredible blend of warming spice, sweetness, and a touch of nuttiness. Drink in the morning or midday for a gentle and sustained energy boost.

Time: 10 minutes

Equipment: Juicer and blender

Yield: Approximately one 16-ounce (475 ml) milk

Ingredients:

1 piece (½ inch, or 1 cm) fresh ginger

1 medium yam

3 pitted medjool dates

½ teaspoon ground turmeric

2 teaspoons (10 g) maca powder

1 cup (235 ml) unsweetened almond milk

¼ teaspoon ground cinnamon

Pinch ground cloves

Pinch ground nutmeg

Pinch ground cardamom

Preparation:

Pass the ginger and yam through a juicer.

Transfer the juice to a blender and add the dates, turmeric, maca, almond milk, cinnamon, cloves, nutmeg, and cardamom.

Blend on high for 20 seconds or until smooth. Enjoy the creamy goodness!

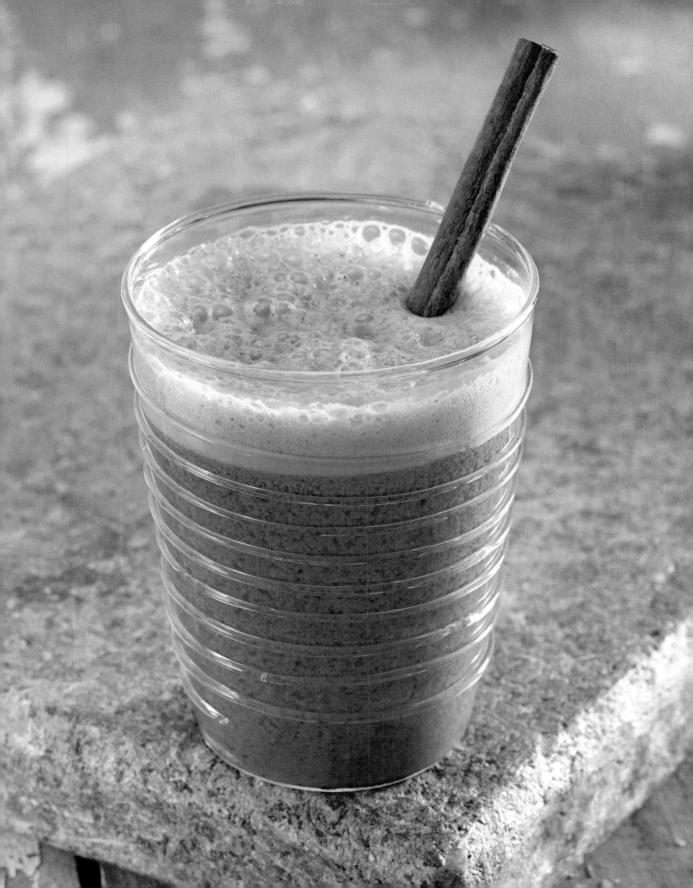

✦MEXI MILK STEAMER✦

Welcome a day in decadence! The rich flavors of cacao, spice, and malt in this hot and creamy creation will lift your libido and mellow your mood while providing a gentle boost of energy. Enjoy this frothy sipper as an excellent alternative to your morning coffee. It provides energy while delivering loads of antioxidants and other nutrients such as magnesium, vitamin A, and prebiotics, which are dietary fibers absorbed from food that support the growth of healthy bacteria. Every sip will deeply nourish you, bring harmony to your body, and set you up for sustained well-being throughout the day.

Time: 10 minutes

Equipment: Small saucepan and milk frother

Yield: Approximately one 12-ounce (355 ml) steamer

Ingredients:

¾ cup (175 ml) unsweetened almond milk

½ cup (120 ml) coconut water

1 tablespoon (6 g) raw cacao powder

1 teaspoon maca powder

1 teaspoon vanilla extract

¼ teaspoon ground cinnamon

⅛ teaspoon cayenne pepper, to taste

1 tablespoon (7 g) yacon or (20 g) maple syrup

Preparation:

Warm the almond milk and coconut water on the stove over medium-high heat. Do not bring to a boil.

Using a milk frother, whip until slightly foamy and then pour into your favorite mug.

Stir in the cacao and maca powders, vanilla, cinnamon, cayenne, and yacon or maple syrup. Enjoy!

✦LOVER SMOOTHIE✦

This drink gets the "lover" name for two reasons. One, its combination of flavors are "lovely," and two, it exhibits aphrodisiac properties as maca delivers nutrients that support hormone regulation and increase sexual desire. You'll love the abundance of sweet and antioxidant-rich strawberries and potassium-balancing banana. Blended with coconut milk, sweet, cooling coconut water, and savory basil, you are sure to fall in love with this delectable blend!

Time: 5 minutes

Equipment: Blender

Yield: Approximately one 20-ounce (570 ml) smoothie

Ingredients:
1 cup (145 g) fresh or (255 g) frozen strawberries
1 small banana
½ cup (120 ml) coconut water
½ cup (120 ml) coconut milk
2 teaspoons (10 g) maca powder
6 large basil leaves

Preparation:
In a blender, combine the strawberries, banana, coconut water, coconut milk, maca powder, and basil.

Blend on high for 20 seconds or until smooth. Be wrapped in bliss!

✦LEMON ROSEMARY FROTH✦

This unexpected blend of ingredients will knock your socks off! It came by way of a lemon rosemary sauce experiment. While I was adding a little of this and a little of that to achieve a savory and citrusy blend to top zucchini pasta, I realized how incredible the medley of flavors could taste if served as a drink. With just a couple tweaks, it was ready for sharing. Lemon juice and zest are detoxifying and support liver health. Ginger will soothe an upset tummy and aid in digestion. Rosemary has nutrients that increase blood flow to the brain, enhancing concentration and contributing to better memory. So next time you have to feel "on," blend up this baby before you head out the door. It can be served hot or cold. If hot, just warm coconut milk over the stove, add all ingredients except ice, and then whip with a milk frother. Mmm mmm!

Time: 5 minutes

Equipment: Blender

Yield: Approximately one 18-ounce (520 ml) froth

Ingredients:

1 lemon, juiced

½ teaspoon lemon zest

1 piece (¼ inch, or 6 mm) fresh ginger, mashed

4 rosemary needles

2 teaspoons (10 g) maca powder

2 tablespoons (32 g) coconut butter

1½ cups (355 ml) light coconut milk

2 tablespoons (13 g) yacon syrup

10 ice cubes

Preparation:

In a blender, combine all the ingredients.

Blend until frothy. Enjoy immediately and say, "Yum!"

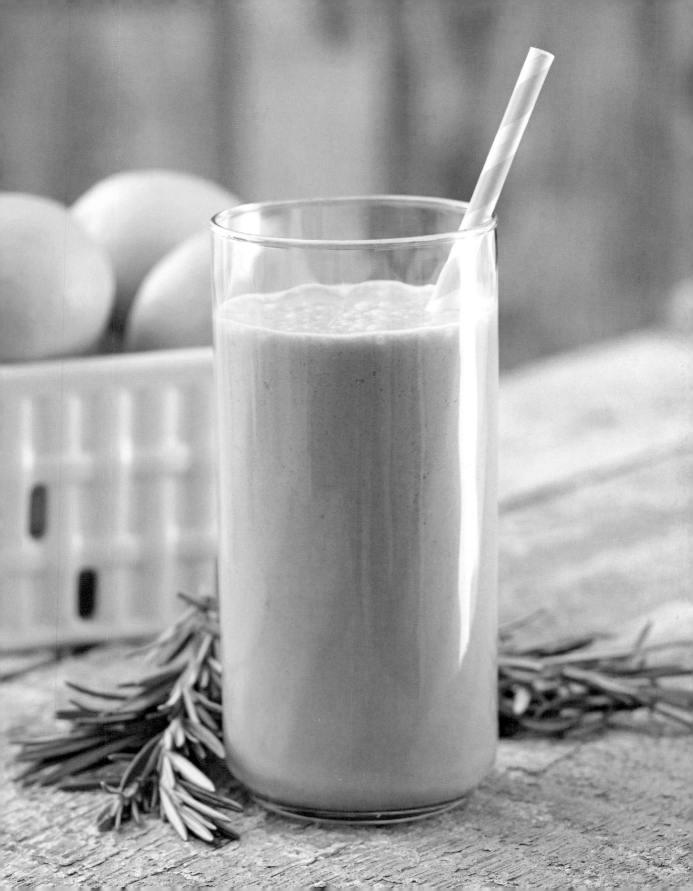

CHAPTER 18

YACON

LOW-GLYCEMIC SWEETENER AND DIGESTIVE AID

FEATURED RECIPES

Calm and Collected Cider

Loving My Greens Juice

Dirty Chai

Racy Root Smoothie

Sweet Maria Smoothie

Yacon, which in the Andean languages translates to "watery root," is known in its native Peruvian land as "ground apple." This root produces an increasingly common sweetener used by rawtarians and vegans but has not yet gained mainstream popularity. The sweet potato–looking tuber has the crunchy texture and relative taste of an apple, which is likely why it was given its ground apple name. Some say the flavor of fresh yacon is similar to watermelon.

Yacon is native to and grows abundantly in South America, where it is commonly eaten fresh and drizzled with lemon or lime juice or tossed with other indigenous sweet delights in exotic fruit salads. Inhabitants of Peru and other South American regions also like to roast, bake, or mash yacon to serve as an accompaniment to meat and beans.

Though commonly called jicama in Ecuador, yacon is not at all related but is actually a member of the sunflower family, which includes the very starchy Jerusalem artichoke, also known as sunchoke. Unfortunately, starches of all kinds get a bad rap for being high on the glycemic index and downright off-limits

for those wanting to lose weight or manage their blood sugar levels. The truth is that not all starchy vegetables and roots are created equal, and yacon is particularly special.

SWEET TUBER BALANCES YOUR BLOOD SUGAR

The syrup and powder of yacon, which both taste similar to molasses, support the balance of your blood sugar levels by not causing them to rise or spike like other common sweeteners do. This tasty and nutritious sugar alternative contains a large amount of fructooligosaccharides (FOS), which are sugar molecules derived from a nondigestible carbohydrate called *inulin*.

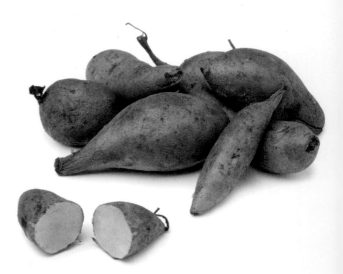

The FOS molecules provide nearly half of yacon's sweet flavor. What's nifty is that we get to experience the sweet taste, but because we do not have a digestive enzyme to hydrolyze FOS, it passes through our digestive tract literally unmetabolized. As a result, the caloric burden of eating yacon is far less than we experience with other sweeteners, and our blood sugar levels go unaffected. Cool, huh?

In a 2009 study conducted by seven researchers at the University San Miguel de Tucumán in Argentina, insulin-resistant obese volunteers were given two doses of yacon syrup each day. At the end of the study, participants demonstrated significantly lower fasting insulin levels. Researchers also noted that their daily intake of yacon syrup produced a significant decrease in body weight, waist circumference, and body mass index.

YACON IS GOOD FOR YOUR GUT

Healthy gut function and frequent stool elimination is essential to our overall health and well-being. This is how we release toxins and waste from the body that can otherwise be stored, putrefy, and promote disease. Yacon supports the health of your digestion, again with the help of FOS.

Because these molecules are not digested in our stomach, they travel to the colon, where they serve as food for the good bacteria that reside there. The bacteria feed on the FOS, multiplying and increasing the population of the good gut bacteria. We want this! Having an abundance of healthy bacteria enhances our immunity, reduces the population of harmful organisms, and increases the frequency of our bowel movements and elimination of toxins.

Sourcing and Care of Yacon

Certified organic yacon syrup and powder can be found online and at most health food stores. Both can be used in a variety of culinary capacities, including as a substitute for high-glycemic sweeteners in baked goods; to sweeten raw desserts, smoothies, and hot and cold cereals; to enhance sauces and dressings; and to mellow the strength of coffee and tea. To achieve the same level of satisfaction as you would get with other sugars, substitute with the equivalent amount of yacon.

Like some other superfoods with incredible health benefits, yacon is not the most inexpensive food. An 8-ounce (225 g) jar of the syrup can range between $11 and $20 depending on the manufacturer. But in my opinion, it is better to pay for high-quality foods to support your health now so you can avoid racking up expensive medical bills later. How sweet of an idea is that?

In a 2008 study led by researcher S. Karger AG at the University Hospital in Basel, Switzerland, five clinicians studied the effect of yacon on colonic transit time. Sixteen volunteers were administered yacon syrup every day in an amount equivalent to about 1 tablespoon (15 ml). Their results showed a significant decrease in waste transit time through the gastrointestinal tract. In addition, stool elimination frequency was increased as well as made more comfortable.

✦CALM AND COLLECTED✦ CIDER

Every system of our body is negatively affected by stress, which increases our susceptibility to illness. That's why it's time we give ourselves permission to take a breather. You won't be able to help but want to take some time out, put your feet up, and sip this calming elixir to release tension. The active ingredient in kava, kavalactone, has soothing properties, promotes nerve and muscle relaxation, and contributes to a sense of emotional well-being. Ginger and cinnamon when mixed with fresh apple juice create a flavor reminiscent of spiced cider and further restore your sense of calm. Not only will this warm and cozy drink make you feel good, its sweet and peppery taste will also dance on your taste buds as it nestles you right into deep relaxation.

Time: 10 minutes

Yield: Approximately one 12-ounce (355 ml) cider

Ingredients:

1 cup (235 ml) fresh-pressed apple juice, heated

1 teaspoon fresh ginger, grated

Pinch ground cinnamon

1 teaspoon fresh lemon juice

1 tablespoon (7 g) yacon syrup

8 drops liquid kava extract (optional for extra calm)

Preparation:

In your favorite mug, add all the ingredients. Stir to combine and bring on the calm.

+LOVING MY GREENS JUICE+

If you just simply can't stand the taste of green juice, please give this one a chance. You just might be surprised at how not green it tastes. The zesty lemon and ginger add some nice zing, and the green taste is cut by the sweetness of yacon and tanginess of green apple. Ginger is anti-inflammatory and good for your gut, kale and lemon are excellent detoxifiers, celery promotes healthy heart function, cucumber tones and brightens your skin, and yacon sweetens without spiking your blood sugar. Doesn't sound so bad right? Bottoms up!

Time: 10 minutes

Equipment: Juicer

Yield: Approximately one 16-ounce (475 ml) juice

Ingredients:

1 piece (½ inch, or 1 cm) fresh ginger

1 medium lemon, peeled, with pith intact

4 kale leaves

4 celery stalks

2 green apples, halved

1 medium cucumber, ends trimmed

2 tablespoons (13 g) yacon syrup

Preparation:

Pass the ginger, lemon, kale, celery, apples, and cucumber through a juicer.

Transfer to a serving glass and stir in the yacon. Enjoy!

✦DIRTY CHAI✦

I enjoy all kinds of chai, but this particular blend is my favorite, not only because it tastes heavenly, but it offers a slow and steady energy boost and is incredibly soothing to digestion. Cloves, cinnamon, fennel, cardamom, and coriander all have gut-nourishing properties that aid digestion. Yerba mate tea contains about 80 mg of caffeine per 1 tablespoon (6 g), but the loads of antioxidants in the tea help slow caffeine absorption, making the stimulant uptake much more of a smooth progression. Yacon is sweet on the tongue, while promoting friendly bacteria to flourish in your gut.

Time: 20 minutes

Equipment: Spice/coffee grinder and French press

Yield: Approximately one 12-ounce (355 ml) chai

Ingredients:

2 cardamom pods

1 whole clove

6 black peppercorns

8 fennel seeds

3 whole coriander seeds

1 tablespoon (6 g) yerba mate loose leaf tea

1 cup (235 ml) hot water (almost boiling)

1 piece (¼ inch, or 6 mm) fresh ginger, peeled, and mashed

¼ teaspoon ground cinnamon

½ cup (120 ml) unsweetened almond milk

1 to 2 tablespoons (7 to 13 g) yacon syrup (to taste)

Preparation:

In a spice or coffee grinder, combine the cardamom, clove, peppercorns, fennel, and coriander. Pulse until you achieve a fine spice blend. Set aside.

In a French press, add the yerba mate leaves, ground spices, and ginger and cover with hot water. Let steep for 15 minutes.

Heat the almond milk and cinnamon on your stove over medium heat until almost boiling. Pour in the tea and heat for one minute.

Pour into your favorite mug, sweeten to taste with yacon syrup, and settle in to tea time!

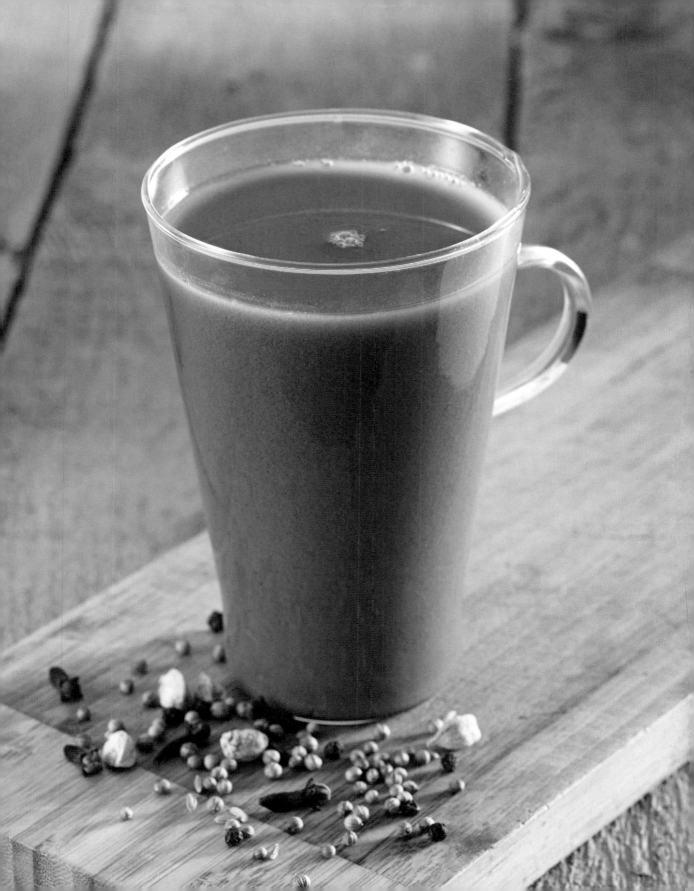

✦RACY ROOT SMOOTHIE✦

I call this smoothie racy root because the base is sweet potato, not an ingredient you normally see in a smoothie but one I just love! Also, its racy reputation comes from the addition of heart-benefiting red hot chili pepper. Why did I use sweet potato? It's deliciously sweet when juiced raw, and it is a powerful anti-inflammatory food. When mixed with immune-boosting Ruby Red grapefruit and sweet coconut water and yacon, the flavor is unique and simply exquisite!

Time: 5 minutes

Equipment: Juicer and blender

Yield: Approximately one 20-ounce (570 ml) smoothie

Ingredients:
½ small red chili pepper (seeds optional)
1 medium Ruby Red grapefruit, peeled, with pith intact
1 medium sweet potato, scrubbed
1 cup (235 ml) coconut water
2 tablespoons (13 g) yacon syrup

Preparation:
Pass the chili pepper, grapefruit, and sweet potato through a juicer in the order specified.

Transfer to a blender and add the coconut water and yacon syrup.

Blend until smooth. Enjoy!

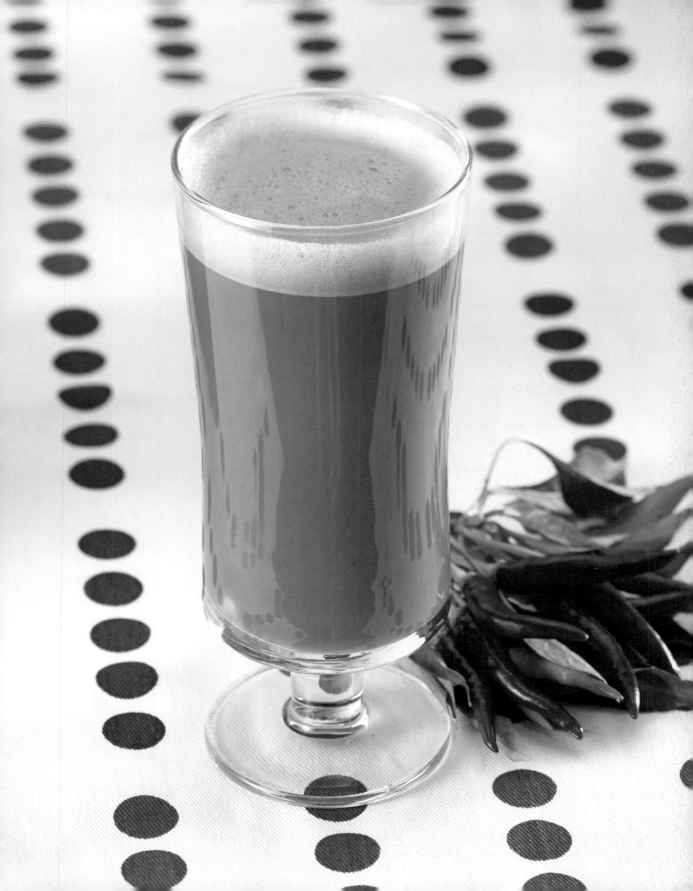

✦SWEET MARIA SMOOTHIE✦

Cilantro—either you love it or you hate it, and if you hate it, I hope to make a fan out of you with this refreshing smoothie recipe. The flavor of cilantro is understated and adds just enough zip to the combination of creamy banana and sweet orange. In addition, cilantro is one of the richest plant sources of vitamin K, your bone nutrient. It also marries harmoniously with fresh lime juice, which adds a little extra pep. Coconut water is cooling to the body and balances your electrolyte levels, and yacon brings all the flavors together as it goes to work on building up your healthy gut army.

Time: 5 minutes

Equipment: Blender

Yield: Approximately one 20-ounce (570 ml) smoothie

Ingredients:
1 small banana
1 cup (235 ml) fresh-pressed orange juice
1 cup (235 ml) coconut water
1 lime, juiced
1 small handful fresh cilantro leaves
2 tablespoons (13 g) yacon syrup

Preparation:
In a blender, combine all the ingredients.

Blend on high for 20 seconds or until smooth. Enjoy!

CHAPTER 19

BEE POLLEN

THE ALLERGY AID

FEATURED RECIPES

Peter Rabbit Smoothie

Allergy Obliterator Smoothie

Fit for a Queen Smoothie

Tropical Sting Smoothie

Purple Pollinator Smoothie

The instinctive reaction to run from or shoo bees away when they buzz by is natural, but you may want to rethink how you relate to them. Bees are vital to our food system. In fact, one-third of our food supply relies on bee pollination in order for crops to grow! Some favorites we wouldn't be able to enjoy without the help of bees are apples, almonds, zucchini, broccoli, tomatoes, kiwi, all berries, coconut, cantaloupe, nectarines, cucumbers, and sunflower seeds. Can you imagine a life without flowers, fresh fruit, and crunchy seeds and nuts? Sounds bleak to me.

ALLEVIATE ALLERGIES WITH POLLEN

The golden granules collected from flowering plants by honeybees are known as bee pollen. As bees travel from one flower to the next, bits of the gathered pollen drop onto neighboring flowering crops. This natural occurrence is called pollination. Not only is bee pollen immensely essential to the flourishing of crops, it has numerous medicinal and holistic healing properties as well.

The nutritional composition of bee pollen is approximately 60 percent carbohydrate, 35 percent protein, 3 percent minerals and vitamins, and 2 percent fatty acids. According to the *Encyclopedia of Healing Foods,* bee pollen is frequently referred to as "nature's most perfect food" because it contains all essential amino acids. The super nutrient also provides vitamins B and C, essential minerals, carotene, plant hormones, and numerous flavonoid molecules. Flavonoids, a group of pigments abundant in bee pollen, have antioxidant, antibacterial, antiviral, antiallergenic, and anti-inflammatory properties.

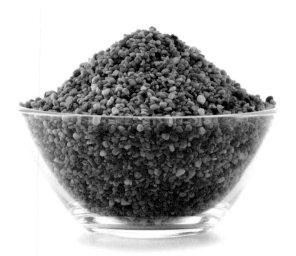

According to Joseph Mercola, DO, in his article "The Use of Bee Pollen as a Superfood," bee pollen can help improve the immune system, calm the nervous system, and help to reduce seasonal allergies. Although it may seem counterproductive to treat seasonal allergies with one of the very substances that may be causing them, pollen, it has been noted that ingesting a small dose of what ails our allergies actually provides defense against seasonal reactions. This technique is the same as that of vaccinations and is called desensitization. It was developed in London at St. Mary's Hospital Medical School after the turn of the century. The treatment involves introducing a small amount of the patient's allergen into the body. Doing so stimulates an antibody response, thus building resistance to allergic reactions.

FIGHT INFECTIONS WITH BEE POLLEN

In a 2005 journal article, six researchers at the Hacettepe University Faculty of Science in Turkey suggested bee pollen might increase production of white blood cells. More white blood cells means improved immune function and protection against disease and infections. In the study *The Effect of Trifolium, Raphanus and Cistus Pollen Grains on Some Blood Parameters and Mesentery Mast Cells,* animal subjects that were fed 60 mg of pollen per day for thirty days demonstrated an increase in lymphocyte levels. Lymphocytes are a type of white blood cell and are the major cellular component of immune response. Think of lymphocytes as soldiers, helping to fight off toxins and health inhibitors. An increased number of lymphocytes means a stronger immune defense, so go on and get some bee pollen!

Sourcing and Care of Bee Pollen

Bee pollen is commonly found in the refrigerated section of your health food market and should be stored in a tightly sealed container to maintain optimal freshness. It should smell and taste fresh, exhibit a deep yellow hue, and not clump or cling together. Stored in the refrigerator, it will remain fresh for up to one year.

If you are consuming bee pollen to help reduce allergy symptoms, only purchase local varieties. This will ensure you are helping to reduce the symptoms of allergies that you are exposed to daily. If you're consuming bee pollen for the first time, start with approximately ⅛ teaspoon to ensure you do not have an adverse* reaction. Slowly increase to no more than 1 teaspoon per day for maintenance.

According to Prescription for Nutritional Healing by Phyllis A. Balch, CNC, approximately 0.05 percent of the population is allergic to bee pollen.

✦PETER RABBIT SMOOTHIE✦

Full of vibrant color and pizzazz, this smoothie is a party in a glass! A combination of creamy banana, spicy ginger, rich cinnamon, and energy-enhancing bee pollen are sure to help you tackle the day or prepare you for a night on the town. If your night got a little too wild, you can also make this beverage first thing in the morning as an enjoyable hangover aid. Ginger is a natural tummy soother, cinnamon helps to regulate blood sugar levels, banana and coconut water both provide electrolyte replenishment, and carrots are a rich source of rejuvenating vitamins and minerals! Talk about a juice that nurtures, not to mention tastes delicious!

Time: 10 minutes

Equipment: Blender

Yield: Approximately one 16-ounce (475 ml) smoothie

Ingredients:

1 cup (235 ml) coconut water

1 cup (235 ml) fresh-pressed carrot juice

1 medium banana

1 piece (½ inch, or 1 cm) fresh ginger, peeled

½ teaspoon ground cinnamon

1 teaspoon local bee pollen

5 to 6 ice cubes

Preparation:

In a blender, combine all the ingredients.

Blend on high for 20 seconds or until smooth. Enjoy immediately and sip slowly.

✦ALLERGY OBLITERATOR✦ SMOOTHIE

Say good-bye to seasonal allergies! By incorporating natural bee pollen and medicinal pau d'arco tea into your daily diet, you can help to reduce allergy symptoms such as puffy and watery eyes, a runny nose, and fatigue. Pau d'arco is a tree native to the rainforests of Central and South America. The bark contains high levels of quercetin, an antioxidant that supports allergy suppression. You can often find the loose bark in the bulk tea isle of your natural food store. It is also available in tea bags and online in either variation. This smoothie provides a serving of allergy reducing bee pollen as well as additional immune-boosting and energy-enhancing ingredients such as blueberries, grapes, and pau d'arco tea. This smoothie is a perfect quick meal to start your day and helps fight allergies all day long.

Time: 30 minutes

Equipment: French press and blender

Yield: Approximately one 20-ounce (570 ml) smoothie

Ingredients:

10 ounces (285 ml) boiling water

1 tablespoon (6 g) pau d'arco tea (loose bark shavings)

½ cup (75 g) red seedless grapes

1 piece (½ inch, or 1 cm) fresh ginger, peeled

½ cup (75 g) fresh or frozen blueberries

1 teaspoon yacon syrup

½ teaspoon local bee pollen

8 ice cubes

Preparation:

Pour boiling water over pau d'arco bark in a French press. Let steep for 15 minutes, strain brewed tea into a mug, and let cool in the refrigerator for 15 minutes.

When the tea is cool, add to a blender along with the rest of the ingredients.

Blend on high for 20 seconds or until smooth. Enjoy immediately and sip slowly.

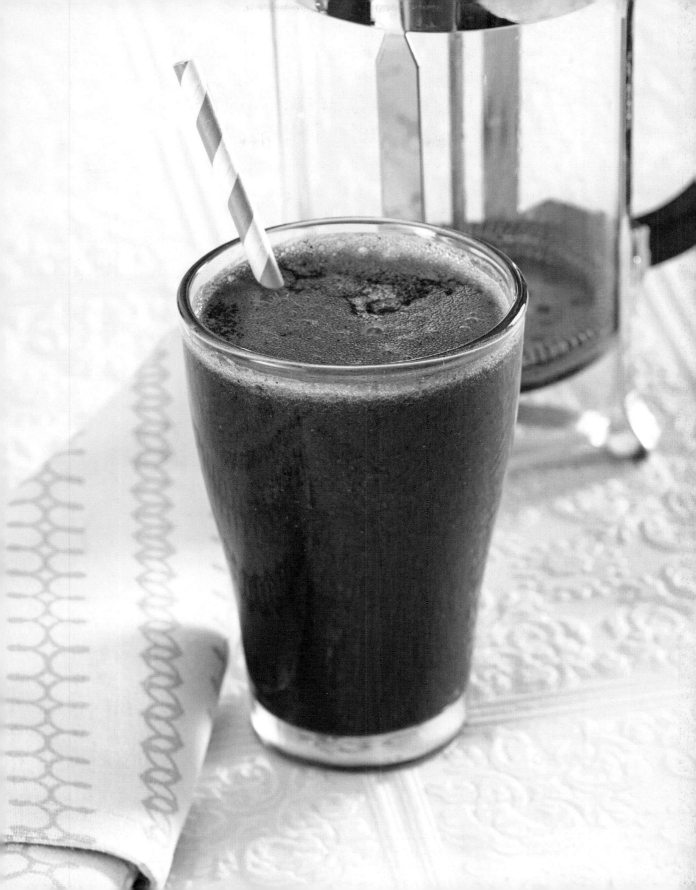

✦FIT FOR A QUEEN✦ SMOOTHIE

To feel like a queen you must sip and nosh like a queen! The superfood ingredient lineup in this sweet and healthful sipper is fit for royalty. You will feel radiant, refreshed, and energized, and your taste buds will be delighted after sipping this royal blend. Kiwi is abundant in antiaging and antioxidant-rich vitamin C (a queen must always look her best). Bee pollen is antibacterial and antiviral, keeping foreign toxins far out of sight and stopping them from getting in the way of your glow! Blended with succulent sweet strawberries, beautifying chia seeds, and creamy almond milk, this smoothie nourishes the body to help you maintain your seat at the throne.

Time: 5 minutes

Equipment: Blender

Yield: Approximately one 20-ounce (570 ml) smoothie

Ingredients:

1 cup (30 g) spinach leaves

½ cup (75 g) fresh or frozen strawberries

1 small kiwi, skin cut away

1 cup (235 ml) unsweetened almond milk

1 tablespoon (7 g) yacon syrup

1 tablespoon (8 g) chia seeds

5 to 6 ice cubes

½ teaspoon local bee pollen

Preparation:

In a high-speed blender, combine the spinach, strawberries, kiwi, almond milk, yacon syrup, chia seeds, and ice.

Blend on high for 20 seconds or until smooth.

Pour into a serving glass and sprinkle with bee pollen.
Enjoy immediately and savor.

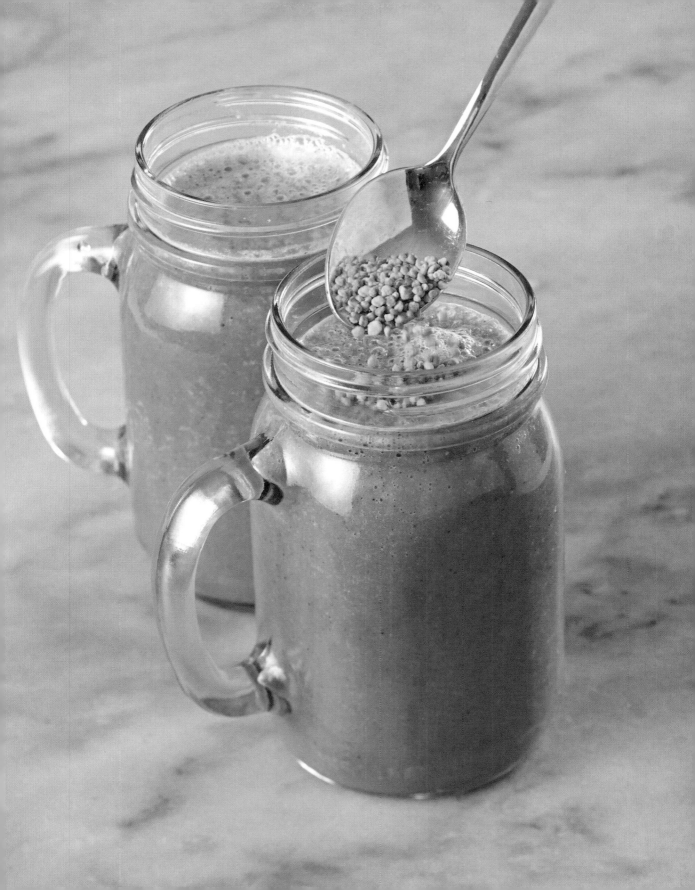

✦TROPICAL STING✦ SMOOTHIE

The flavors of this smoothie will teleport you to the tropics. Made with sweet, tangy, and succulent ingredients, it deserves a tiny umbrella and wedge of pineapple. Also, it is a cinch to make and may just become a staple of yours to sip on any time. The main attraction of this delicious blend is fresh-brewed yerba mate. This South American tea has a robust flavor, boasts twenty-four vitamins and minerals, fifteen amino acids, is abundant in antioxidants, and stimulates energy without leaving you feeling jittery. Blended together with sweet and refreshing pineapple juice, creamy banana, coconut, and bee pollen, this smoothie is fit for the islands. Aloha!

Time: 5 minutes

Equipment: Blender

Yield: Approximately one 20-ounce (570 ml) smoothie

Ingredients:
1 cup (235 ml) brewed yerba
    mate iced tea
1 cup (235 ml) fresh pineapple
    juice, not from concentrate
1 medium banana
¼ cup (20 g) shredded
    unsweetened coconut
½ teaspoon local bee pollen
5 to 6 ice cubes

Preparation:
In a blender, combine all the ingredients.

Blend on high for 20 seconds or until smooth. Enjoy immediately and savor!

✦PURPLE POLLINATOR✦ SMOOTHIE

One sip of this smoothie and you will forever fall in love with medjool dates! Not only are they rich in natural sweetness, they have bounds of nourishing properties. They contain an abundance of fiber, high levels of essential minerals such as potassium, magnesium, copper, and manganese. Combined with creamy banana, antioxidant-rich blueberries, peppery ginger, calcium-filled almond milk, and our beloved bee pollen, this smoothie is one that you will love, and it will love you back!

Time: 5 minutes

Equipment: Blender

Yield: Approximately one 20-ounce (570 ml) smoothie

Ingredients:
½ cup (75 g) fresh or frozen blueberries

1 piece (¼ inch, or 6 mm) fresh ginger, peeled

2 cups (475 ml) unsweetened almond milk

2 pitted medjool dates

1 medium banana

5 to 6 ice cubes

½ teaspoon local bee pollen

Preparation:
In a high-speed blender, combine the blueberries, ginger, almond milk, dates, banana, and ice.

Blend on high for 20 seconds or until smooth. Pour into a serving glass and sprinkle with bee pollen. Enjoy immediately and savor.

CHAPTER 20

ALOE VERA

SKIN SOOTHER AND TUMMY TAMER

FEATURED RECIPES
Skin Soother Juice
Coco-Vera Fresca
Aloe Envy Smoothie
Blackberry Breeze Smoothie
Piña Pleaser Juice

It is likely you have slathered aloe vera gel on a stinging sunburn and experienced cooling relief of irritated skin. The succulent plant of North African origin contains two distinct compounds that make it an effective anti-inflammatory and skin-nourishing serum. The polysaccharides (carbohydrates comprised of a number of sugar molecules) in the gel support skin growth and repair. Glycoproteins, proteins that also contain sugar molecules, reduce inflammation. In addition, aloe vera gel has antimicrobial and antibacterial properties that help fight inflammatory skin conditions such as acne. Vitamins C and E are naturally present in the gel and improve the texture and support hydration of our skin, which is why aloe vera is sometimes a prominent ingredient in skin care products.

Did you know that the nourishing qualities of aloe go beyond the superficial layers of your skin?

Research has shown that this medicinal plant can slow or inhibit cancer cell division and drinking the juice of the aloe vera plant works as a natural laxative to move toxins through your gut and out of your body.

SLATHER ON ALOE TO INHIBIT CANCEROUS SKIN CELL DIVISION

Medical professionals have discovered the gel of the aloe leaf can actually inhibit the process of cancerous skin cell division. In September 2012, researchers from the University of Belgrade School of Medicine confirmed that aloe-emodin, a constituent of aloe, is effective in inhibiting cell division of human skin cells that had been treated with radiation. In the study, the aloe-emodin stopped the proliferation process and confirmed aloe's ability to halt the progression of tumor formation resulting from sun radiation.

Another study found similar results. Researchers from South Korea's Gachon University of Medicine

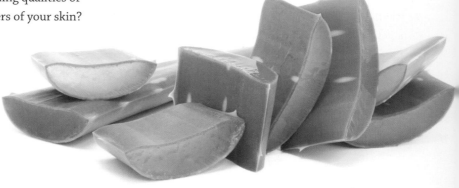

and Science found that aloe-emodin stimulated a genetic change within the cancerous cells that not only halted their growth, but also induced death of the tumor cells. So if you find yourself in the unfortunate circumstance of getting crispy from too much sun exposure, replenish your skin cells with pure, chemical-free aloe gel. By "pure" I mean as close to the inner plant gel as possible if not straight from the plant. Avoid use of the blue- or green- tinted goops you can find at the drug store. The preservatives and chemicals added to make the gel more appealing can be harmful and may negate aloe's positive effects. According to the book *A Consumer's Dictionary of Cosmetic Ingredients*, synthetic colors and pigments may cause irritation and skin sensitivity.

ALOE JUICE IS GOOD FOR YOUR GUT

Inner leaf aloe vera gel and juice are nourishing health tonics that support a healthy balance of good gut bacteria. By promoting regular and complete bowel movements, your intestines can remove toxins and better maintain the right amount of beneficial microorganisms. A healthy balance of these good gut guys is essential to strong immunity and contributes to the effective breaking down and absorption of nutrients.

Another way aloe juice supports the health of your gut is by keeping yeast growth in check. Yeast is present in all of our intestines but can overgrow and cause candida growth to proliferate. Candida is a yeastlike fungus that if grown in excess can contribute to intestinal discomfort and infections such as athlete's foot, vaginal yeast infections, and even oral thrush, a yeast infection of the mouth. Constipation and slow elimination transit times fuel the growth of yeast and cause a disproportionate number to flourish. Some common symptoms of yeast overgrowth include gas, bloating, sugar cravings, itchy skin, rashes, and constipation.

A component of the aloe leaf pulp, referred to as the latex, contains anthraquinone, which gives aloe its laxative-like qualities. In addition, these compounds are helpful in keeping your GI tract clean and microorganisms in balance. They also help to loosen toxins that tend to collect in the colon due to lack of healthy elimination. This action flushes built-up waste residue and gently expels it from your body.

In a 1991 study conducted at Soroka Medical Center in Beersheba, Israel, thirty-five men and women who suffered from chronic constipation were randomly selected to receive capsules containing a blend of celadin, aloe vera, and psyllium. At the end of the twenty-eight-day trial, those subjects who received the capsules, as opposed to those who were given a placebo, experienced more frequent bowel movements, their stools were softer, and the need for other laxatives was reduced.

BOOST IMMUNITY WITH ALOE JUICE

Aloe juice contains a complex carbohydrate known as acemannan, which has antiviral and antibacterial properties. In 2010, five researchers at the Department of Pharmaceutics, MAEER's Maharashtra Institute of Pharmacy in Pune, India, discovered that when an ointment consisting of aloe vera gel, neem, and curcumin was applied to subjects with skin infections, they demonstrated prominent antifungal and some antibacterial activity and accelerated healing.

PRACTICE MODERATION WHEN INGESTING ALOE

It's true—you can get too much of a good thing. The maximum recommended intake of aloe vera juice and gel is no more than 2 ounces (60 ml) per day. An excess of this amount can cause unpleasant abdominal cramping and diarrhea. Additionally, aloe should be used only as needed, not consumed regularly.

Prolonged use can result in skin rash or hives and a dependency on the food supplement for regular bowel movements. Mayo Clinic states on its website that those with heart and kidney disease or those who suffer from electrolyte imbalance should use caution when ingesting aloe vera products to avoid the risk of reduced potassium levels.

Sourcing and Care of Aloe Vera

Aloe vera's production is largely unregulated, putting the burden on you to ensure you are purchasing the highest-quality product available. First and foremost, avoid all aloe products that have been treated with dyes or fragrance. Only buy certified organic gel and juice and products proudly wearing the International Aloe Science Council (IASC) seal of approval. Check the label to ensure aloe vera is the only ingredient.

When looking to buy ingestible juices, only buy those that are manufactured from the inner leaf gel, not the whole leaf, as some people experience extreme abdominal discomfort when consuming the latter. Aloe for internal consumption should be stored in the refrigerator. The juice and gel is best when used within thirty days of opening. You may also opt to purchase the common aloe plant sold at garden stores and nurseries, which is excellent to have in the kitchen in case of a burn incident. As needed, snip or break off a small segment of the succulent and squeeze the fresh gel directly on your wound. You can also apply the pure gel to sunburns, rashes, or acne breakouts to reduce redness, inflammation, and discomfort.

Eating the clear, jellylike substance of fresh aloe leaves is considered safe. To eat the whole leaf is not recommended, however, as it contains a compound called latex, which contains laxative-like qualities that has raised safety concerns.

✦SKIN SOOTHER JUICE✦

Our complexion can always benefit from greater clarity and glow.
Nourish your dermis from the inside by sipping on this sweet, tangy, and
refreshing skin tonic. Aloe vera reduces redness and inflammation and
supports elimination of toxins. Green grapes can help reduce constipation.
As a result, you eliminate more frequently, encouraging a cleaner body
and more vibrant skin. Lemon has detoxifying qualities and radishes are
abundant in water and aid in the hydration of your skin. They also contain
disinfectant properties that reduce skin blemishes and breakouts.

Time: 5 minutes

Equipment: Juicer

Yield: Approximately one
16-ounce (475 ml) juice

Ingredients:
1 medium lemon, peeled,
   with pith intact

3 medium red radishes

1 cup (150 g) green grapes

1 medium semisweet apple
   (such as Gala), halved

1 medium cucumber, ends trimmed

⅛ cup (28 g) inner leaf aloe
   vera gel or juice

Preparation:
Pass the lemon, radishes, grapes,
apple, and cucumber through
a juicer in the order specified.

Transfer to a serving glass and
stir in the aloe gel or juice. Enjoy
immediately and sip slowly.

✦COCO-VERA FRESCA✦

With a little time, you can make this incredibly satisfying and nourishing fresca that's rich in omega-3 fatty acids, fiber, minerals, and digestive-aiding properties. Perfect as a post-workout or hot yoga refresher, coconut water rehydrates the body and supports electrolyte balance, and chia seeds provide protein to aid in muscle recovery. Working from the inside out, aloe gel and juice nourish skin that may have become dehydrated and dry from excessive perspiration.

Time: 1 hour (includes chill time)

Equipment: 16-ounce (475 ml) glass jar

Yield: Approximately one 16-ounce (475 ml) fresca

Ingredients:

4 ounces (120 ml) coconut water, plus 8 ounces (235 ml)

2 teaspoons (5 g) chia seeds

⅛ cup (28 g) inner leaf aloe vera gel or juice

Preparation:

In a glass jar, combine 4 ounces (120 ml) coconut water with the chia seeds. Let rest for ten minutes. Stir and rest ten minutes more.

Add the remaining coconut water and aloe gel or juice. Stir to combine and then refrigerate until chilled, about 40 minutes. Enjoy!

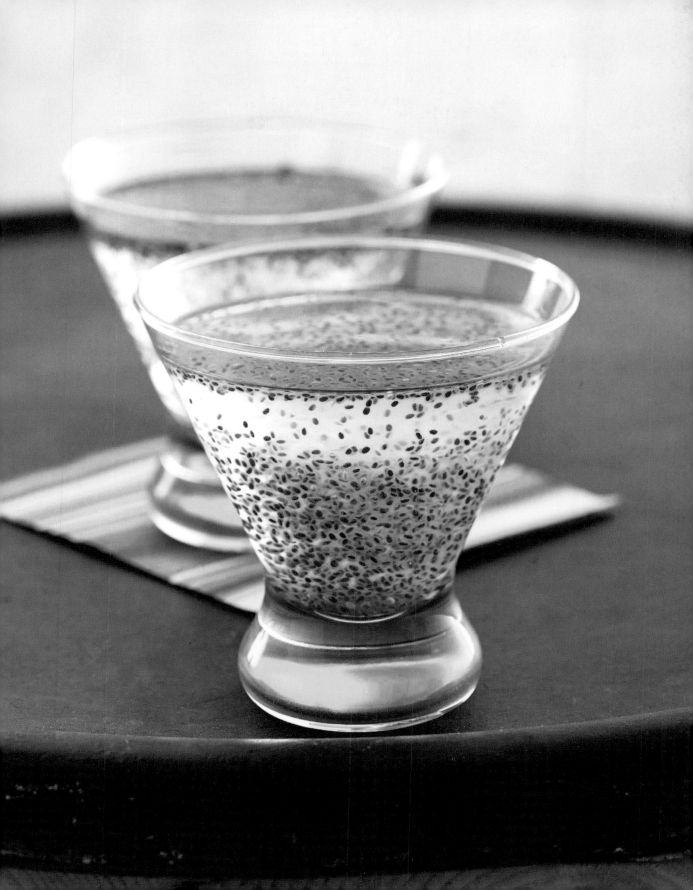

✦ALOE ENVY SMOOTHIE✦

This creamy coconut delight is filling and nutritionally balanced. Avocado adds richness and texture while delivering an abundance of fiber and healthy fats. Coconut milk contains lauric acid, an antibacterial and anti-fungal compound that promotes immunity. Dates sweeten the smoothie and deliver blood-strengthening iron, and kale is rich in vitamin K, a vital nutrient for bone development and strength. Pretty impressive nutrient lineup, don't you think?

Time: 5 minutes

Equipment: Blender

Yield: Approximately one 20-ounce (570 ml) smoothie

Ingredients:

3 large kale leaves, de-ribbed and chopped

½ medium avocado

2 cups (475 ml) light coconut milk

2 tablespoons (13 g) coconut flakes

4 pitted medjool dates

⅛ cup (28 g) inner leaf aloe gel or juice

Preparation:

In a blender, combine all the ingredients.

Blend on high for 20 seconds or until smooth. Enjoy immediately and sip slowly.

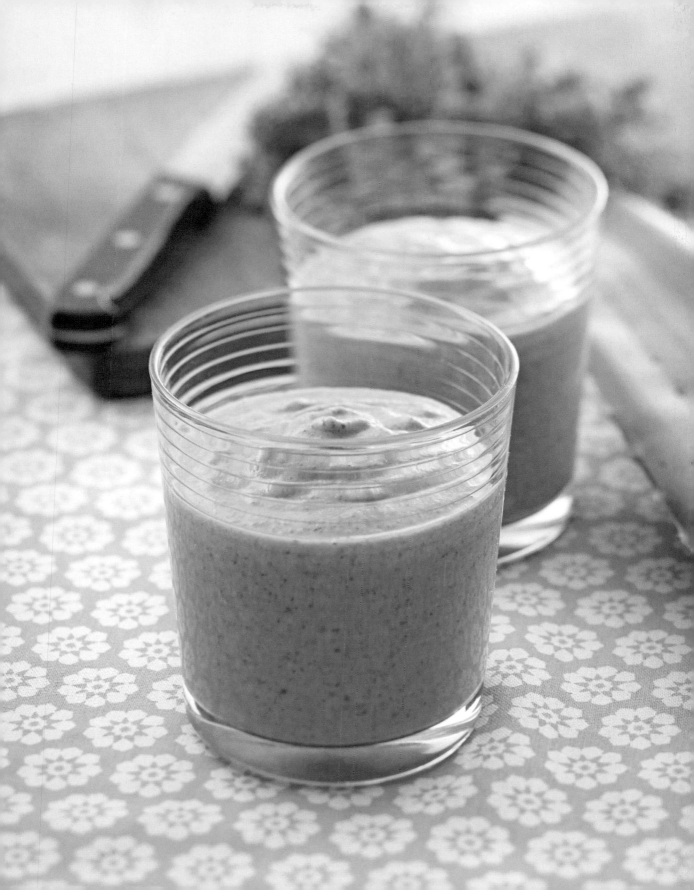

✦BLACKBERRY BREEZE✦ SMOOTHIE

When blackberries are in season, there is almost no other fruit that tastes more luscious. Sweetened with low-glycemic yacon and hydrating coconut water, their natural tang is enhanced and balanced in this smoothie. Stomach-soothing mint adds vibrancy and freshness to this cool and delicious blend, and coconut oil boosts energy and revs your metabolism for optimum caloric burn.

Time: 5 minutes

Equipment: Blender

Yields: Approximately one 20-ounce (570 ml) smoothie

Ingredients:
½ cup (75 g) fresh blackberries

6 to 8 mint leaves

⅛ cup (28 g) inner leaf aloe vera gel or juice

1 tablespoon (14 g) coconut oil

2 tablespoons (13 g) yacon syrup

Pinch sea salt

2 cups (475 ml) coconut water

6 to 8 ice cubes

Preparation:
In a blender, combine all the ingredients.

Blend on high for 20 seconds or until smooth. Enjoy immediately and sip slowly.

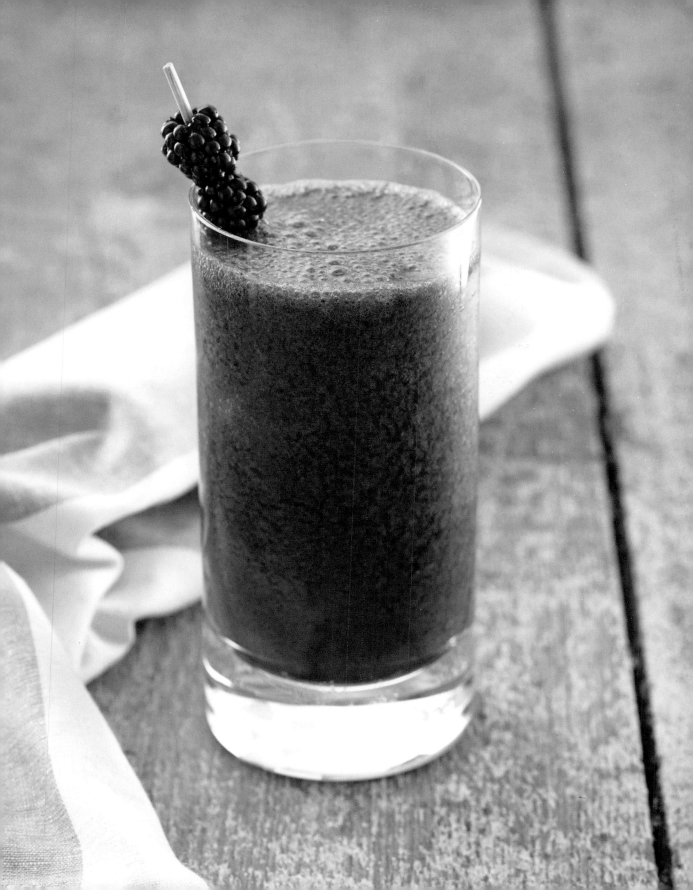

✦PIÑA PLEASER JUICE✦

Simple and refreshing, this enzyme-rich juice supports gut health by enhancing digestive activities. Fresh pineapple is frothy and sweet and compatible with succulent orange. Both are fans of cooling coconut water, and all team up perfectly with immune-boosting and digestion-enhancing aloe.

Time: 5 minutes

Equipment: Juicer

Yield: Approximately one 16-ounce (475 ml) juice

Ingredients:

2 cups (330 g) fresh pineapple

2 medium navel oranges, skin cut away, with pith intact

½ cup (118 ml) coconut water

⅛ cup (28 g) inner leaf aloe vera gel or juice

Preparation:

Pass the pineapple and oranges through a juicer.

Transfer to a large glass and stir in the coconut water and aloe gel or juice. Enjoy immediately and sip slowly.

RESOURCES

SUPERFOOD POWDERS AND SUPPLEMENTS
Navitas Naturals
www.navitasnaturals.com

Kiva Tea Bar & Spa
http://kivateaspa.com

Sunfood
www.sunfood.com

AFA
www.e3live.com

ALOE PRODUCTS
Lily of the Desert
www.lilyofthedesert.com

BULK SPICES, HERBS, AND TEAS
Frontier Co-op
www.frontiercoop.com

Kalustyan's
www.kalustyans.com

JUICERS AND BLENDERS
Two-part juicer
www.norwalkjuicers.com

Masticating juicer
www.amazon.com

Centrifuge juicer
www.breville.com

Vitamix high power blender
www.vitamix.com

RECOMMENDATIONS
Coconut oil
www.nutiva.com

Matcha green tea powder
www.mercola.com

Yerba Mate loose leaf tea
www.guayaki.com

Sunwarrior Classic Protein
www.sunwarrior.com

Manitoba Hemp Protein Powder
www.manitobaharvest.com

Probiotics, vitamins, and minerals
www.megafood.com

Water filters
www.multipure.com

OTHER RESOURCES
Balanced Raw (by the author)

HappyCow vegetarian food finder
www.happycow.net

VegNews magazine
www.vegnews.com

Haute Health (author's site)
www.hautehealthnow.com

Dr. Joseph Mercola
www.mercola.com

Be Well Buzz
www.bewellbuzz.com

Institute for Integrative Nutrition (IIN)
www.integrativenutrition.com

NaturalNews Network
www.naturalnews.com

The pH Miracle Alkaline-Acid Food Chart
www.phmiracleliving.com/
t-food-chart.aspx

Care2 Community
www.care2.com

My Crazy Sexy Life
www.mycrazysexylife.com

REFERENCES

PART 1: SUPER FRUITS

Chapter 1: Goji—The "Red Diamond" of Nutrition

Harunobu Amagase, PhD, Dwight M. Nance, PhD, "A Randomized, Double-Blind, Placebo-Controlled, Clinical Study of the General Effects of a Standardized Lycium barbarum (Goji) Juice, Gochi," The Journal of Alternative and Complementary Medicine, May 2008. Accessed September 4, 2013, http://online.liebertpub.com/doi/abs/10.1089/acm.2008.0004.

Harunobu Amagase, PhD, Dwight M. Nance, PhD, "Lycium barbarum increases caloric expenditure and decreases waist circumference in healthy, overweight men and women: Pilot study," American College of Nutrition, October 2011. Accessed September 4, 2013, www.ncbi.nlm.nih.gov/m/pubmed/22081616.

Chapter 2: Camu Camu: Vitamin C Superstar

James May, PhD, "Vitamin C Transport and Its Role in the Central Nervous System," Sub-cellular Biochemistry, 2012. Accessed September 4, 2013, www.ncbi.nlm.nih.gov/pubmed/22116696.

T. Inoue, H. Komoda, T. Uchida, K. Node, "Tropical Fruit Camu-Camu (Myciaria dubia) Has Anti-oxidative and Anti-Inflammatory Properties," Journal of Cardiology, October 2008. Accessed September 4, 2013, www.ncbi.nlm.nih.gov/pubmed/18922386.

Chapter 3: Maqui: Disease-Fighting Antioxidants

Alternative Medicine. Cathy Wong, ND, CNS, "Maqui: What You Need to Know about Maqui," updated June 26, 2013. Accessed September 15, 2013, http://altmedicine.about.com/od/herbsupplementguide/a/Maqui.htm.

S. Miranda-Rottmann, A. A. Aspillaga, D. D. Pérez, L. Vasquez, A. L. Martinez, F. Leighton, "Juice and Phenolic Fractions of the Berry Aristotelia Chilensis Inhibit LDL Oxidation in vitro and Protect human endothelial cells against oxidative stress," Journal of Agricultural and Food Chemistry, December 2002. Accessed September 15, 2013, www.ncbi.nlm.nih.gov/pubmed/12475268.

A. Basu, M. Rhone, T. J. Lyons, "Berries: Emerging Impact on Cardiovascular Health," Nutrition Reviews, March 2010. Accessed September 4, 2013, www.ncbi.nlm.nih.gov/pubmed/20384847.

Izabela Konczak, Wei Zhang, "Anthocyanins—More than Nature's Colours," Journal of Biomedicine and Biotechnology, December 2004. Accessed September 4, 2013, www.ncbi.nlm.nih.gov/pmc/articles/PMC1082903/.

Chapter 4: Lucuma: The "Gold of the Incas"

Natural Nutritional Health. Barry Lutz, "Lucuma Powder—Nutritious Low Glycemic Natural Sweetener," August 8, 2012. Accessed September 15, 2013, www.naturalnutritionalhealth.com/healthy-foods-recipes/lucuma-powder-nutritious-low-glycemic-natural-sweetener/.

Living in Peru. Mariella Balbi, "Kingdom of the Egg-fruit, Lucuma," October, 2004. Accessed September 4, 2013, http://archive.peruthisweek.com/gastronomy/features-1036.

Sacred Chocolate. David Wolfe, "The Agave Blues," 2010. Accessed September 4, 2013, www.sacredchocolate.com/docs/sacredpdf/agave-blues-david-wolfe.pdf.

Chapter 5: Golden Berries: Protein-Packed Powerhouses

BMC Cancer. Hsueh-Wei Chang, Yang-Chang Wu, "4β-Hydroxywithanolide E from *Physalis peruviana* (golden berry) inhibits growth of human lung cancer cells through DNA damage, apoptosis and G2/M arrest," February 2010. Accessed September 5, 2013, www.biomedcentral.com/1471-2407/10/46.

Open Access Scientific Reports. Mónika Valdenegro, "The Effects of Drying Processes on Organoleptic Characteristics and the Health Quality of Food Ingredients Obtained from Goldenberry Fruits (*Physalis Peruviana*)," January 2013. Accessed September 5, 2013, www.omicsonline.org/scientific-reports/srep642.php.

Chapter 6: Cacao: Magnesium Wonder Fruit

Weil. Andrew Weil, MD, "Q & A Library," August 2011. Accessed September 5, 2013, www.drweil.com/drw/u/QAA400995/Is-Cocoa-as-Healthy-as-Dark-Chocolate.html.

AARP. Candy Sagon, ed., "Harvard Study: Dark Chocolate Can Lower Your Blood Pressure," March 2011. Accessed September 5, 2013, www.aarp.org/health/medical-research/info-03-2011/dark-chocolate-can-help-lower-your-blood-pressure.html.

The Nibble. Peter Rot, MD, "High Percentage Cacao Chocolate," June 2013. Accessed September 5, 2013, www.thenibble.com/reviews/main/chocolate/high-percentage-cacao-chocolate.asp.

PART 2: SUPER SEEDS AND NUTS

Chapter 7: Chia: Aztec Warrior Superfood

Centers for Disease Control and Prevention, Heart Disease, updated September 2013. Accessed September 5, 2013, www.cdc.gov/heartdisease/.

Cleveland Clinic Wellness. Roxanne B. Sukol, MD, MS, Brenda Powell, MD, "Chia Seeds Supplement Review." Accessed September 5, 2013, www.clevelandclinicwellness.com/Features/Pages/Chia-Seeds.aspx.

Chapter 8: Hemp: The Heart-Healthy Superfood

Mercola. Hans R. Larsen, MSc, ChE. "Omega-3 Oils: The Essential Nutrients." Accessed September 5, 2013, www.mercola.com/beef/omega3_oil.htm.

ANewDayANewMe. "Dr Oz: Omega 3 and Omega 6. All Omegas Are Not Created Equal and May Be Harmful to Your Health." Accessed September 5, 2013, www.anewdayanewme.com/dr-oz-omega-3-and-omega-6-all-omegas-are-not-created-equal-and-may-be-harmful-to-your-health.

University of Maryland Medical System. Steven D. Ehrlich, NMD, "Omega-6 Fatty Acids," updated June 17, 2011. Accessed September 5, 2013, http://umm.edu/health/medical/altmed/supplement/omega6-fatty-acids.

The National Center for Biotechnology Information. F. H. Chilton, L. L. Rudel, J. S. Parks, J. P. Arm, M. C. Seeds, "Mechanisms by which Botanical Lipids Affect Inflammatory Disorders," *The American Journal of Clinical Nutrition*, February 2008. Accessed September 5, 2013, www.ncbi.nlm.nih.gov/pubmed/18258646.

University of Maryland Medical System. "Gamma-Linolenic Acid," July, 2011. Accessed September 5, 2013, http://umm.edu/health/medical/altmed/supplement/gammalinolenic-acid.

Chapter 9: Flax: Brain-Boosting Super Seed

Healthsmart. Beatrix Hon, "Flaxseed," January 2009. Accessed September 5, 2013, http://traditionalacupuncture.files.wordpress.com/2011/07/flaxseed-article.pdf.

National Health Association. Jeff Novick, MS, RD, "Flax: Just the Facts Please," 2002. Accessed September 5, 2013, www.healthscience.org/Articles/flax_article.htm.

G. K. Paschos, F. Magkos, D. B. Panagiotakos, V. Votteas, A. Zampelas, "Dietary Supplementation With Flaxseed Oil Lowers Blood Pressure in Dyslipidaemic

Patients," *European Journal of Clinical Nutrition*. October 2007. Accessed September 5, 2013, www.ncbi.nlm.nih.gov/pubmed/17268413?dopt=Abstract.

David Schardt, "Just the Flax," *Nutrition Action Healthletter*. December 2005. Accessed September 5, 2013, www.cspinet.org/nah/12_05/flax.pdf.

SheKnows. Michele Borboa, MS, "Matcha: The Healthiest Green Tea," September 2009. Accesed September 17, 2013, www.sheknows.com/health-and-wellness/articles/811034/matcha-the-healthiest-green-tea.

Deborah Josefson, "Fishy Diet Could Help Prevent Alzheimer's Disease," *BMJ* (*British Medical Journal*). August 2003. Accessed September 5, 2013, www.ncbi.nlm.nih.gov/pmc/articles/PMC1150899/.

Chapter 10: Sacha Inchi: Omega-3 Power Seed

Dr Oz. "10 Simple Rules to Lose 5 Pounds," July 3, 2012. Accessed September 15, 2013, www.doctoroz.com/videos/10-simple-rules-lose-5-pounds.

Chapter 11: Coconut: The Super Fat

Melissa Clark, "Once a Villain, Coconut Oil Charms the Health Food World," *The New York Times*. March 2011. Accessed September 5, 2013, www.nytimes.com/2011/03/02/dining/02Appe.html?pagewanted=all&_r=0.

M. Sachs, J. Von Eichel, F. Asskali, "Wound Management with Coconut Oil in Indonesian Folk Medicine," Der Chirurg; Zeitschrift für alle Gebiete der operativen Medizen. April 2002. Accessed September 5, 2013, www.ncbi.nlm.nih.gov/pubmed/12063927.

M. L. Assuncão, H. S. Ferreira, A. F. dos Santos, C. R. Cabral, Jr, T. M. Florêncio, "Effects of Dietary Coconut Oil on the Biochemical and Anthropometric Profiles of Women Presenting Abdominal Obesity," *Lipids*. July 2009. Accessed September 5, 2013, www.ncbi.nlm.nih.gov/pubmed/19437058.

J. O. Hill, J. C. Peters, D. Yang, T. Sharp, M. Kaler, N. N. Abumrad, H. L. Greene, "Thermogenesis in Humans During Overfeeding with Medium-Chain Triglycerides," *Metabolism: Clinical and Experimental*. July 1989. Accessed September 5, 2013, www.ncbi.nlm.nih.gov/pubmed/2739575.

Mercola. Joseph Mercola, DO, "Here's the Smarter Oil Alternative I Recommend to Replace Those Other Oils in Your Kitchen." Accessed September 5, 2013, http://products.mercola.com/coconut-oil/.

PART 3: SUPER PLANTS

Chapter 12: Kale—The Mega Flavonoid Super Green

National Cancer Institute. "Fact Sheet: Antioxidants and Cancer Prevention," reviewed July 2004. Accessed September 5, 2013, www.cancer.gov/cancertopics/factsheet/prevention/antioxidants.

American Cancer Society. "Cancer Facts & Figures 2013." Accessed September 5, 2013, www.cancer.org/research/cancerfactsstatistics/cancerfactsfigures2013/ index.

American Cancer Society, "Diet and Physical Activity: What's the Cancer Connection?" updated January 24, 2013. Accessed May 18, 2013. www.cancer.org/cancer/cancercauses/dietandphysicalactivity/diet-and-physical-activity.

W. J. Blot, J. Y. Li, P. R. Taylor, et. al., "Nutrition Intervention Trials in Linxian, China: Supplementation With Specific Vitamin/Mineral Combinations, Cancer Incidence, and Disease-Specific Mortality in the General Population," *Journal of the National Cancer Institute*. September 1993. Accessed September 5, 2013, www.ncbi.nlm.nih.gov/pubmed/8360931.

Chapter 13: Spirulina: Nature's Detoxifier

MedlinePlus. "Protein in Diet," updated May 2011. Accessed September 5, 2013, www.nlm.nih.gov/medlineplus/ency/article/002467.htm.

IIMSAM. L. P. Loseva, I. V. Dardynskaya, "Spirulina—Natural Sorbent of Radionucleides," September 1993. Accessed September 5, 2013, www.iimsam.org/publications_and_reports.php.

Smartmicrofarms. Robert Henrikson, "Earth Food Spirulina," 2009. Accessed September 5, 2013, www.smartmicrofarms.com/PDF.cfm/EarthFood Spirulina.pdf.

Spirulina Bahamas. M. Misbahuddin, A. Z. Islam, S. Khandker, Ifthaker-Al-Mahmud, N. Islam, Anjumanara, "Effects of Spirulina—Heavy Metals," *Clinical Toxicology*, 2006. Accessed September 5, 2013, http:// spirulinabahamas.com/Spirulina_Bahamas/Spirulina_ Scientific_documentation__Heavy_metals.html.

Chapter 14: Chlorella: The Vitality Plant

Bio+Sources. Bernard Jensen, D.O., C.N., "Chlorella: Jewel of the East." Accessed September 5, 2013, www.bio-sources.com/chlorellabenefits.

Bio+Sources. Dr. David Steeblock, BS, MSC, DO, "Chlorella Natural Medicinal Algae." Accessed September 15, 2013, www.bio-sources.com/ chlorellabenefits.

Natural News. Mike Adams, "Cleanest Sources for Chlorella Revealed: Natural News Publishes Metals Contamination Test Results for World's Most Famous Superfood," February 2013. Accessed September 5, 2013, www.naturalnews.com/039145_chlorella_ heavy_metals_lab_tests.html.

Chapter 15: Wheatgrass: The Oxidative Stress Buster

Jan Ziegler, "It's not easty being green: chlorophyll being tested," *Journal of the National Cancer Institute.* (January 4, 1995) 87(1):11.

Chapter 16: AFA: Blue-Green Algae: The Immune-Boosting Energizer

Algae-World. Gabriel Cousens, MD, "Microalgae: First & Finest Superfood," *Body Mind Spirit Magazine,* May 1995. Accessed September 5, 2013, www.algae-world. com/algae40.html.

David Wolfe, "AFA Super Blue Green Algae: Primordial Food," in *Superfoods: The Food and Medicine of the Future.* (Berkeley, CA: North Atlantic Books, 2009), 123–137.

Hippocrates Health Institute. "Blood Builders." Accessed September 5, 2013, www.hippocratesinst. org/well-being/blood-builders.

Why Algae. G. S. Jensen, D. I. Ginsberg, P. Huerta, M. Citton, C. Drapeau, "Consumption of *Aphanizomenon flos-aquae* has Rapid Effects on the Circulation and Function of Immune Cells in Humans," *Journal of the American Nutraceuticals Association,* 2000. Accessed September 5, 2013, http://whyalgae.com/ blue-green-algae-research/afa-and-immunity/.

Stem Cell Nutrition. John Taylor, PhD, "Anti-cancer and Anti-virus Studies." Accessed September 15, 2013, http://usafatech.com/Research_BS3O.html.

Weil. "Facts about Vitamin B12, updated October 2012. Accessed September 5, 2013, www.drweil.com/ drw/u/ART02810/facts-about-vitamin-b.

Chapter 17: Maca: The Peruvian Super Plant

C. M. Dording, L. Fisher, G. Papakostas, A. Farabaugh, S. Sonawalla, M. Fava, D. Mischoulon, "A Double-Blind, Randomized, Pilot Dose-Finding Study of Maca Root (L. meyenii) for the Management of SSRI-Induced Sexual Dysfunction," *CNS Neuroscience and Therapeutics.* Fall 2008. Accessed September 5, 2013, www.ncbi.nlm.nih.gov/pubmed/18801111.

G. F. Gonzales, A. Córdova, K. Vega, A. Chung, A. Villena, C. Góñez, S. Castillo, "Effect of Lepidium meyenii (MACA) on Sexual Desire and Its Absent Relationship With Serum Testosterone Levels in Adult Healthy Men," *Andrologia.* December 2002. Accessed September 5, 2013, www.ncbi.nlm.nih.gov/ pubmed/12472620.

NaturoDoc. Garry P. Gordon, MD, "Maca as an anti-aging herb for men and women." Accessed September 5, 2013, www.naturodoc.com/library/nutrition/ maca.htm.

Chapter 18: Yacon: Low-Glycemic Sweetener and Digestive Aid

S. Genta, W. Cabrera, N. Habib, J. Pons, I.M. Carillo, A. Grau, S. Sánchez, "Yacon Syrup: Beneficial Effects on Obesity and Insulin Resistance in Humans," *Clinical Nutrition*. April 2009. Accessed September 5, 2013, www.ncbi.nlm.nih.gov/pubmed/19254816.

A. G. Karger, M. Geyer, I. Manrique, L. Degen, C. Beglinger, "Effect of Yacon (*Smallanthus sonchifolius*) on Colonic Transit Time in Healthy Volunteers," *Digestion*. September 2008. Accessed September 5, 2013, www.ncbi.nlm.nih.gov/pubmed/18781073.

Chapter 19: Bee Pollen: The Allergy Aid

Michael T. Murray, Joseph E. Pizzorno, and Lara Pizzorno, *The Encyclopedia of Healing Foods*. (New York: Atria, 2005).

Mercola. Joseph Mercola, DO, "The Use of Bee Pollen as a Superfood," July 2013. Accessed September 5, 2013, www.mercola.com/article/diet/bee_pollen.htm.

Dürdane Kolankaya, Hakan Şentürk, Ash Özkök Tüylü, Sibel Hayretdağ, Güldeniz Selmanoğlu, Kadriye Sorkun. "The Effect of *Trifolium*, *Raphanus*, and *Cistus* Pollen Grains on Some Blood Parameters and Mesentery Mast Cells," December 2005. Accessed September 5, 2013, www.znaturforsch.com/ac/v61c/s61c0421.pdf.

Phyllis A. Balch, *Prescription for Nutritional Healing*. (New York: Avery, 2010).

Chapter 20: Aloe Vera: Skin Soother and Tummy Tamer

Today I Found Out. "Is Aloe Vera Really Good for Your Skin," January 2013. Accessed September 5, 2013, www.todayifoundout.com/index.php/2013/01/is-aloe-vera-really-good-for-your-skin/.

D. Popadic, E. Savic, Z. Ramic, V. Djordjevic, V. Trajkovic, L. Medenica, S. Popadic, "Aloe-Emodin Inhibits Proliferation of Adult Human Keratinocytes In Vitro," *Journal of Cosmetic Science*. September 2012. Accessed September 5, 2013, www.ncbi.nlm.nih.gov/pubmed/23089351.

GreenMedInfo. Case Adams, ND, "Research Finds Aloe Vera May Prevent and Treat Skin Cancer," December 2012. Accessed September 5, 2013, www.greenmedinfo.com/blog/research-finds-aloe-vera-may-prevent-and-treat-skin-cancer.

Ruth Winter, *A Consumer's Dictionary of Cosmetic Ingredients*. (New York: Three Rivers Press, 2009).

H. S. Odes and Z. Madar, "A Double-Blind Trial of a Celandin, Aloe Vera and Psyllium Laxative Preparation in Adult Patients With Constipation," *Digestion*. 1991. Accessed September 5, 2013, www.ncbi.nlm.nih.gov/pubmed/1800188.

Abhijeet Pandey, Jui V. Jagtap, Aditi A. Patil, Richa N. Joshi, B. S. Kuchekar, "Formulation and Evaluation of Anti-Bacterial and Anti-Fungal Activity of a Herbal Ointment Containing *Aloe-vera*, *Azadirachta indica* and *Curcuma- longa*," *Journal of Chemical and Pharmaceutical Research*. 2010. Accessed September 5, 2013, http://jocpr.com/vol2-iss3-2010/JOCPR-2010-2-3-182-186.pdf.

Mayo Clinic. Aloe (Aloe vera), updated September 1, 2012. Accessed September 15, 2013, www.mayoclinic.com/health/aloe-vera/NS_patient-aloe/DSECTION=safety.

WebMD. "Aloe." Accessed September 5, 2013, www.webmd.com/vitamins-supplements/ingredient mono-607-ALOE.aspx?activeIngredientId=607&activeIngredientName=ALOE.

International Aloe Science Council, www.iasc.org.

INDEX

ABOUT THE AUTHOR

Tina Leigh, CHHC, RYT, founder of Haute Health and author of *Balanced Raw*, is an inspiring and compassionate transformative health practitioner, yoga instructor, and therapeutic chef. She affirms there is not a one-size-fits-all approach to nutrition and well-being. She has a unique ability to weave the principles of Ayurveda and plant-based eating with culinary art that attracts a varied clientele. It is through years of experience, deep empathy, and a devotion to conscious living that she's able to guide those she works with through their unique journeys to whole-body transformation.

Tina is also the creator of the ABC Lifestyle—a commitment to Always Be Cleansing. She also has developed The Eater's Detox—a seven-day food-strong cleanse program.